Midlife and Older Adults and HIV: Implications for Social Service Research, Practice, and Policy

Midlife and Older Adults and HIV: Implications for Social Service Research, Practice, and Policy has been co-published simultaneously as *Journal of HIV/AIDS & Social Services*, Volume 3, Number 1 2004.

Midlife and Older Adults and HIV:
Implications for Social Service Research, Practice, and Policy

Cynthia Cannon Poindexter, PhD, MSW
Sharon M. Keigher, PhD, ACSW
Editors

Midlife and Older Adults and HIV: Implications for Social Service Research, Practice, and Policy has been co-published simultaneously as *Journal of HIV/AIDS & Social Services*, Volume 3, Number 1 2004.

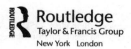

Routledge
Taylor & Francis Group
New York   London

Midlife and Older Adults and HIV: Implications for Social Service Research, Practice, and Policy has been co-published simultaneously as *Journal of HIV/AIDS & Social Services*,™ Volume 3, Number 1 2004.

First pubished by

The Haworth Press, Inc., 10 Alice Street, Binghamton, NY 13904-1580 USA

This edition published 2012 by Routledge

Routledge
Taylor & Francis Group
711 Third Avenue
New York, NY 10017

Routledge
Taylor & Francis Group
2 Park Square, Milton Park
Abingdon, Oxon OX14 4RN

Cover design by Kerry Mack

Library of Congress Cataloging-in-Publication Data

Poindexter, Cynthia Cannon, 1954-
Midlife and older adults and HIV: implications for social services research, practice, and policy / Cynthia Cannon Poindexter, Sharon M. Keigher.
p. cm.
"Co-published simultaneously as Journal of HIV/AIDS & Social Services, Volume 3, Numbers 1 2004."
Includes bibliographical references and index.
ISBN 0-7890-2645-7 (hard cover : alk. paper) – ISBN 0-7890-2646-5 (soft cover : alk. paper)
1. AIDS (Disease) in old age. I. Keigher, Sharon Marie, 1947- II. Title.
RA643.8.P65 2004
618.97' 69792–dc22
2004009663

Midlife and Older Adults and HIV: Implications for Social Service Research, Practice, and Policy

CONTENTS

BRIDGING RESEARCH AND PRACTICE

ABOUT THE EDITORS

Cynthia Cannon Poindexter, MSW, PhD, has been a human services practitioner for 28 years, the last 17 of which have been dedicated to the HIV field. She has taught graduate social workers at the University of Illinois at Chicago, Boston University, and Fordham University, where she is currently Associate Professor. She has been a trainer for the S.C. AIDS Training Network, the Southeast AIDS Education and Training Center, the Midwest AIDS Training and Education Center, the New England AIDS Education and Training Center, the NASW HIV Spectrum Project, the Massachusetts Department of Public Health HIV Division, and the HIV/AIDS Service Administration of New York City.

Sharon M. Keigher, PhD, MA, is Professor in the Helen Bader School of Social Welfare at the University of Wisconsin, Milwaukee. Her interests include funding for human services, Medicaid, welfare, international comparative social policy, health aspects of social problems, homelessness, and inequality. Since 1999 she has been Co-Principal Investigator on an in-depth, Longitudinal Study of Women Living with HIV. Dr. Keigher was Editor-in-Chief of *Health & Social Work* (1998-2002). She co-edited *Aging & Social Work: Changing Landscapes,* and authored *Housing Risks and Homelessness Among the Urban Elderly* as well as over 40 articles and book chapters. She chaired the Social Research Policy & Practice section of the Gerontological Society of America (1997-99).

Introduction

This book represents a milestone. It is our first topical collection to address one of the many emerging needs in the field of HIV/AIDS social services. We are grateful to Cynthia Cannon Poindexter and Sharon M. Keigher, for this timely and relevant volume that sheds new light on the unique issues facing HIV patients over age 50.

At the beginning of the HIV pandemic, the impact of the disease on older adults was seldom considered. However, as many of the authors in this volume describe, HIV-affected older adults are impacted in many ways and their unique challenges warrant our increased attention. Today, an estimated 11 percent and 15 percent of Americans infected with HIV are over age 50. Social service providers have faced many new challenges with addressing the needs of older adults living with HIV. In addressing these challenges, HIV service providers have borrowed heavily from gerontological service delivery. Such concepts as continuum of care, case management, family-based care, psychosocial assessment, addressing stigma and multiple losses, not to mention co-morbidities of various sites all were borrowed, consciously or unconsciously, from the aging service network among others. In past years, older adults were often forgotten in our design of prevention and risk reduction programs; however, there is an emergence of professional literature and intervention designs aimed specifically at the aging population. The challenges as well as emerging solutions are both addressed in this collection.

Dr. Poindexter and Dr. Keigher have compiled a collection rich with valuable resource information, current research findings, innovative conceptual models and program ideas to address the HIV epidemic within the aging population. We thank the authors for all their contributions and for producing the first of what we hope are many enlightening and beneficial publications on critical topics concerning HIV/AIDS and social services.

Nathan L. Linsk and Dorie J. Gilbert
Co-Editors

[Haworth co-indexing entry note]: "Introduction." Linsk, Nathan L., and Dorie J. Gilbert. Co-published simultaneously in *Journal of HIV/AIDS & Social Services* (The Haworth Press) Vol. 3, No. 1, 2004, pp. 1; and: *Midlife and Older Adults and HIV: Implications for Social Service Research, Practice, and Policy* (ed: Cynthia Cannon Poindexter, and Sharon M. Keigher) The Haworth Press, Inc., 2004, pp. 1. Single or multiple copies of this article are available for a fee from The Haworth Document Delivery Service [1-800-HAWORTH, 9:00 a.m. - 5:00 p.m. (EST). E-mail address: docdelivery@haworthpress.com].

http://www.haworthpress.com/web/JHASO
Digital Object Identifier: 10.1300/J187v03n01_01

OVERVIEW

Inclusion of "Older" Adults with HIV

As demographers project a significant increase in HIV among older persons in the decades ahead, the need for increasingly vigorous HIV prevention, outreach, and services to older adults is already upon us. This thematically-focused publication, brings a gerontological perspective to HIV practice and policy. Already in the third decade of the HIV pandemic, with egregious health disparities still reflected in the incidence and prevalence of this devastating disease, middle-aged and older adults with HIV are an age-cohort (among several particularly vulnerable sub-populations) still largely excluded from public attention and HIV services.

From the beginning of the HIV pandemic, consistently 10 to 12 percent of persons diagnosed with AIDS [end-stage HIV disease] have been over the age of fifty.[1] By 1998 the proportionate increase in AIDS was greater in adults over 50 than among young adults (Centers for Disease Control and Prevention [CDC], 1998). By the end of 2001, more than 90,000 persons (11 percent of all U.S. persons diagnosed with AIDS) had become ill with AIDS at or beyond age 50, excluding persons over 50 who had asymptomatic HIV and those diagnosed with AIDS at younger ages who are now 50 or over (CDC, 2002). As is the case in all age groups, there have been steady increases in females, Blacks,

Cynthia Cannon Poindexter, PhD, MSW, is Associate Professor at Fordham University Graduate School of Social Service.

Sharon M. Keigher, PhD, ACSW, is Professor at the Helen Bader School of Social Welfare, University of Wisconsin Milwaukee.

[Haworth co-indexing entry note]: "Overview." Poindexter, Cynthia Cannon, and Sharon M. Keigher. Co-published simultaneously in *Journal of HIV/AIDS & Social Services* (The Haworth Press) Vol. 3, No. 1, 2004, pp. 3-8; and: *Midlife and Older Adults and HIV: Implications for Social Service Research, Practice, and Policy* (ed: Cynthia Cannon Poindexter, and Sharon M. Keigher) The Haworth Press, Inc., 2004, pp. 3-8. Single or multiple copies of this article are available for a fee from The Haworth Document Delivery Service [1-800-HAWORTH, 9:00 a.m. - 5:00 p.m. (EST). E-mail address: docdelivery@haworthpress.com].

Digital Object Identifier: 10.1300/J187v03n01_02

and Latinos and Latinas among these midlife and older persons with HIV (CDC, 2002).

Despite the known presence of HIV in the 50-plus population, HIV prevention campaigns rarely feature midlife and older adults, perpetuating a myth that this age group is not at risk for infection. HIV service systems have tended to under-serve midlife and older persons, and local aging service systems have rarely sought out persons with HIV. Social service workers in the HIV field tend to know little about aging, and gerontological social services rarely address either the public or service recipients directly about HIV. We should be doing better.

EARLY AGENDA SETTING FOR HIV, AGING, AND SOCIAL WORK

This volume is an extension of social work advocacy efforts that started early in the HIV epidemic when few resources were available to practitioners working with midlife and older persons. In New York in the late 1980s, social workers Karen Solomon, Gregory Anderson, Rose Dobrof and Marie Nazon, and nurse Kathleen Nokes began community-based efforts to advocate for this population by helping form the New York AIDS and Aging Task Force (now the New York Association of HIV Over Fifty). In 1989 Tulane University social work professor Gary Lloyd called for more coalition building between the HIV and Aging networks to meet the needs of HIV-positive elders (Lloyd, 1989). Also in 1989 Riley, Ory, and Zablotsky's *AIDS in an Aging Society* was published, a pioneer academic work examining the needs of infected and affected elders. In 1994 *Families in Society*'s special issue on social work and HIV included an article highlighting aging as a social work HIV-related issue (Linsk, 1994). In 1996 a coalition of groups sponsored at Hunter College in New York the first conference on HIV and aging. Due to the urging of Vincent Delgado, a Florida social worker, the conference convened a general meeting to establish a national organization to advocate for HIV issues affecting older populations. From this conference grew the National Association of HIV Over Fifty (NAHOF), an organization still jointly lead by older consumers and service providers together bridging the worlds of HIV and gerontology.

In the mid-1990s an HIV Interest Group began meeting regularly at the annual scientific meetings of the Gerontological Society of America. In 2002 this group spearheaded a special HIV-focused issue of the *Journal of Mental Health and Aging*. Having brought HIV practice concerns to a gerontological journal, that group next sought to bring a gerontological perspective to an HIV practice journal. The *Journal of HIV/AIDS & Social Services: Research, Practice and Policy*, which had been recently developed through work of the National Social Work AIDS Network (NSWAN) at the Annual Conference on Social Work and HIV, seemed to be an appropriate venue. Co-editors for a thematic issue related to aging and HIV were soon recruited and called for papers on research, policy, prevention, and practice concerns relevant to midlife and older persons with HIV.

Today scholarship is expanding rapidly on the complex realities of persons over 50 living with HIV. In June 2003 an authoritative anthology of scholarship appeared in the *Journal of Acquired Immune Deficiency Syndromes* (volume *33*, Supplement 2), having grown out of a national symposium convened by several federal agencies including the National Institute on Aging of the National Institutes of Health. Charles Emlet has edited and augmented the special issue of the *Journal of Mental Health and Aging (2004)* that has been released as a book. In it Zablotsky and Kennedy's 2004 overview of the history of epidemiology and research on HIV in midlife and older adults is an excellent resource. Another new book, Nichols et al. (2003), *Aging with HIV: Psychological, Social, and Health Issues,* is reviewed by Daphne Joslin in this issue. A growing bibliography on HIV and aging can be found at the NAHOF website (www.hivoverfifty.org).

EMERGING AWARENESS OF THE GRAYING OF HIV

Today's research on HIV and aging is sprinkled throughout the scholarly journals of widely disparate disciplines and professions, available to enrich the perspective and understanding of social service practitioners. Both integration and specialization is needed in the professional literature to raise awareness of the special needs and assets of older adults infected by HIV. As Zablotsky and Kennedy (2004) point out, over the past 15 years there has been so much epidemiology and research generated on living with HIV at midlife and older that it is not useful to claim that we know nothing about this group–rather, we know a great deal about the wide diversity found in this population. Researchers have clearly documented the wide diversity found in this older population. Using qualitative, quantitative, and mixed methods, many researchers are illuminating the particular confluence of factors confronting persons dealing with both HIV and aging. This volume is a modest but important contribution to that literature and to ongoing advocacy efforts.

The challenge facing the social work profession now is to disseminate new knowledge on the intersection of this disease at this life stage efficiently to practitioners in both aging and HIV. More practitioners need to collaborate with clinical researchers to build our empirical literature, developing more effective and relevant prevention and service interventions, demonstrating and evaluating them, identifying the key indicators of effective programs, and selling them to policy makers.

While highlighting older persons with and vulnerable to HIV who are 50 and older, we acknowledge the unique risks facing other age groups as well, including their rights to preventive public health and primary care, medical treatment, social care, and freedom from oppression. We ask simply that *no* group with HIV be ignored, neglected, or excluded from public compassion and responsibility. Excluding any age, ethnic, or cultural group from attention simply jeopardizes the health of society at large. HIV advocacy is already too vulnerable to divisive interests and every infected human being is equally deserving of attention and assistance.

THIS COLLECTION

The articles here add to both our knowledge base and our research agenda, identifying issues that are not yet fully understood. Emlet examines social service utilization, finding that midlife and older persons with HIV tend to rely more heavily on the HIV network than the Aging Network. He challenges both networks to integrate care and coordinate efforts for persons eligible for services in both systems. He hints at the hybrid organizational forms, matrices, and cross-population case-management that may well become standard practice in another decade. Winningham and associates address the vulnerability of midlife and older African American women in the rural South. They surveyed the women's perceptions of their partner's risk for HIV and their own ability to negotiate for safer sex. They found the women did not accurately perceive their vulnerability to HIV, and they remind service providers not to succumb to that same mistake. Keigher, Stevens, and Plach report on the health, social, and economic factors shaping the everyday experiences of fifty-something HIV-positive women in Wisconsin. Examining the stories of nine such women, the authors question whether "successful aging," as traditionally defined, is even possible for women in the face of HIV's financial, physical, and emotional costs.

Also examining "successful aging," Vance and Robinson examine some recent medical breakthroughs that reveal the interface of neurophysiology, behavioral health, and social stress, reminding us that little of the ameliorative care social services provide would be effective without the costly advances of medical science and pharmacology. In the "Bridging Research and Practice" article, Neundorfer and associates describe a pilot study of a behavioral intervention designed to help midlife and older persons with HIV compensate for cognitive declines. Their study suggests that, with support, people with mild cognitive losses can still follow complex medication regimes to maintain functioning and independence. As more efficient telecommunications technology and effective psycho-education protocols like this develop, social workers will surely be expected to incorporate them into standard practice.

This collection has a high level of scholarship, but we wanted to also have creative and community-based perspectives. We have included a book review, some personal narratives, and resources for networking. Daphne Joslin reviews the latest book on HIV and aging. Poindexter presents interviews with 6

HIV-positive persons over 50, giving voice to some real people behind the statistics. Finally, NAHOF provides an additional resource list for service providers and groups that link HIV and aging issues.

This publication, read primarily by social workers and other service providers in the HIV field, calls for renewed attention by practitioners to advocacy, service, education, and policy interventions on behalf of midlife and older persons with HIV. With every possible source of oppression felt by midlife and older persons with HIV–xenophobia, addiction phobia, homophobia, sexism, ageism, HIV stigma, racism, mental health stigma, and classism–discrimination must be addressed in all its forms. Dealing with any one of these "whammies" is overwhelming, but the combination can be disastrous. The needs are great for targeted outreach, education, and services; culturally competent care; and systems linkages. AIDS Service Organizations must continue to form partnerships with the Aging Network, and social workers must more intensely collaborate with other disciplines to develop relevant and effective services for midlife and older persons with HIV. Social workers, who have always helped health care providers recognize cutting edge issues, must know the relevant co-morbidity factors as midlife and older persons try to manage symptoms stemming from HIV, medication side effects, conditions associated with aging, or any combination of all these.

In addition to Dr. Linsk and Dr. Gilbert, we wish to thank the following experts from social work, HIV, and/or gerontology who reviewed manuscripts: Julie Bach, Roslyn Chernesky, Charles Emlet, Larry Gant, Irene Gutheil, Linda Harootyan, Nancy Kropf, Regina Kulys, Helen Land, Sally Mason, Kathy Nokes, Andrea Rae, Lisa Razzano, James Skinner, Darryl Wheeler, and Diane Zablotsky. Their labors, along with those of the contributors, make this book relevant, authoritative, and well worth reading.

Cynthia Cannon Poindexter, PhD, MSW
Sharon M. Keigher, PhD, ACSW

NOTE

1. When CDC began monitoring reported incidence and prevalence of AIDS in 1982, age was reported as: under 25, 25 to 44, 44 to 49, and over 49. That is why people who talk and write about HIV and aging tend to use age 50 as the beginning of that group, although no one views 50 as "old" in any traditional sense. Due to pressure from activists, CDC now further categorizes HIV and AIDS reporting by these age groups: 45-54, 55-64 and 65-plus (CDC, 2002, p. 14). Incrementally we are learning about HIV and AIDS in this population. It is hoped that soon the age group between 70 and 100 will be reported in detail as well.

REFERENCES

Centers for Disease Control and Prevention [CDC] (1998). AIDS among persons aged greater than or equal to 50 years, United States, 1991-1996. *Morbidity and Mortality Weekly, 47*(02), 21-27.

Centers for Disease Control and Prevention [CDC] (2003). AIDS cases in adolescents and adults, by age, United States, 1994-2000. *HIV/AIDS Surveillance Supplemental Report, 9*(1), 1-25.

Centers for Disease Control [CDC] (2002). HIV/AIDS Surveillance Report, Vol. 14, p. 14.

Emlet, C.A. (ed) (2004). *HIV/AIDS and older adults: Challenges for individuals, families, and communities.* NY: Springer Publishing.

Journal of Acquired Immune Deficiency Syndromes, 33 (Supplement 2) (2003).

Journal of Mental Health and Aging, 8(4) (special issue) (2002).

Linsk, N.L. (1994). HIV and the elderly. *Families in Society, 75*, 362-372.

Lloyd, G.A. (1989). AIDS and elders: Advocacy, activism, & coalitions. *Generations, Fall*, 32-35.

Nichols, J.E., Speer, D.C., Watson, B.J., Watson, M.R., Vergon, T.L., Vallee, C., & Meah, J.M. (2003). *Aging with HIV: Psychological, Social, and Health Issues.* Elsevier Science.

Riley, M. W., Ory, M. G., & Zablotsky, D. (Eds.), *AIDS in an aging society.* New York: Springer Publishing.

Zablotsky, D. & Kennedy, M. (2004). Assessing the progress and promise of research on midlife and older adults and HIV/AIDS. In Emlet, C. A. (Ed). *HIV/AIDS and older adults: Challenges for individuals, families, and communities.* NY: Springer Publishing.

Knowledge and Use
of AIDS and Aging Services
by Older, HIV-Infected Adults

Charles A. Emlet, PhD, MSW

SUMMARY. Older adults living with HIV/AIDS require a complex array of services. Such needs can be addressed both by the service network developed for HIV as well as the network developed for older persons. This study of adults, age 50 and over with HIV/AIDS (N = 41), compared the knowledge and use of services commonly available from the HIV network as well as the aging network. The study sample had similar knowledge of HIV services and services designed for older adults. These individuals, however, used a significantly higher number of services provided through the HIV network (mean of 2.61 services) compared to the aging network (mean of .68 services). Predictors for service use varied across systems. While the primary predictor of HIV service use was awareness, Medicaid eligibility and living arrangements were predictive of use of services from the aging network. *[Article copies available for a fee from The Haworth Document Delivery Service: 1-800-HAWORTH. E-mail address: <docdelivery@haworthpress.com> Website: <http://www.HaworthPress.com> © 2004 by The Haworth Press, Inc. All rights reserved.]*

Charles A. Emlet, PhD, is Assistant Professor of Social Work and a Hartford Scholar in Geriatric Social Work at the University of Washington, Tacoma.

The assistance of Sondra Perdue, Dr. P.H., in the analysis of the data was greatly appreciated.

This research was supported through a grant from the John A. Hartford Foundation and the Hartford Social Work Faculty Scholars Program.

[Haworth co-indexing entry note]: "Knowledge and Use of AIDS and Aging Services by Older, HIV-Infected Adults." Emlet, Charles A. Co-published simultaneously in *Journal of HIV/AIDS & Social Services* (The Haworth Press) Vol. 3, No. 1, 2004, pp. 9-24; and: *Midlife and Older Adults and HIV: Implications for Social Service Research, Practice, and Policy* (ed: Cynthia Cannon Poindexter, and Sharon M. Keigher) The Haworth Press, Inc., 2004, pp. 9-24. Single or multiple copies of this article are available for a fee from The Haworth Document Delivery Service [1-800-HAWORTH, 9:00 a.m. - 5:00 p.m. (EST). E-mail address: docdelivery@haworthpress.com].

KEYWORDS. Aging, HIV/AIDS, older adults, service utilization, Ryan White, Older Americans Act

An important focus of research in various areas of health and social services has been of service utilization. A major purpose in studying service utilization is based on the premise that service planning and programming can be greatly enhanced through improved knowledge of the characteristics of persons using specific services (Harel, Noelker, & Blake, 1985). Service utilization research has historically sought to determine social factors and personal characteristics that influence the use of services.

Researchers in the area of HIV/AIDS have acknowledged the importance of examining service use in order to plan and organize care. As noted by Crystal and Sambamoorthi (1998), as treatment for HIV continues to improve, larger numbers of individuals will live into their 50s and beyond, increasing the importance of understanding their needs and use of services. While a number of studies have examined service utilization among older persons with HIV/AIDS, many of these studies compare use across populations (younger and older) and examine a wide variety of services including hospitalizations, outpatient medical care, and community-based services including case management (Emlet, 1998; Crystal, LoSasso, & Sambamoorthi, 1999; London, LaBlanc & Aneshensel, 1998; Turner, Kelly, & Ball, 1989; Turner, McKee, Fanning, & Markson, 1994; Fritsch, 2001). The results of these studies are mixed. Crystal, LoSasso, and Sambamoorthi (1999) found persons age 55 or older had hospital stays lasting 8.25 days longer than 25-year-olds. The same study, however, noted that although hospitalizations were longer, older persons had fewer hospitalizations than their younger counterparts. Turner and colleagues (1989) found that those aged 45 and older with AIDS experienced longer hospital stays even after controlling for severity of illness. Several studies, however, have documented older persons using lesser amounts of services than younger persons. Turner et al. (1994) found patients older than age 50 less likely to be hospitalized during the five months after AIDS diagnosis. Emlet (1993) found older persons less likely than their younger counterparts to use emotional support services targeted at persons with HIV, and Fritsch (2001) found older Canadians with HIV to access fewer health and medical services and fewer social organizations than a younger comparison group. London, LeBlanc, and Aneshensel (1998) found older age to be associated with a decreased likelihood to initiate case management services. Recently, Emlet and Berghuis (2002) found difference in service use between younger and older adults with HIV/AIDS associated with the need for community-based care, such as home delivered meals, physical therapy, and adult day health care. Differences appear to be related to maintaining independence and stress the importance of aging in place.

Increasingly, social workers, researchers, and other health professionals are recognizing that older persons living with HIV/AIDS may access services through various systems of care. The Ryan White Comprehensive AIDS Resources Emergency (CARE) Act of 1990 (PL101-381), and the Older American's Act of 1965 are two systems of care that can potentially provide services to older adults with HIV/AIDS. These two acts both provide federal funding for services delivered at the local level. The purpose of this paper is to: (1) explore awareness of HIV and aging services among HIV-infected older adults; (2) determine the extent to which older HIV-infected adults access services from each system; and (3) examine the characteristics associated with their knowledge and service use.

SYSTEMS OF CARE

For older adults living with HIV/AIDS, care and services can be obtained from multiple sources including AIDS service organizations (ASOs) as well as the *aging network* (including programs funded under the Older Americans Act (OAA)). The primary mission of most ASOs is to serve people living with HIV/AIDS and/or to provide HIV prevention/education services. ASOs can be important to older adults as ASOs possess expertise in developing and delivering HIV-specific, culturally sensitive programs (Topolski, Gotham, Klinkenberg, O'Neill, & Brooks, 2002). Similarly, a wide array of services designed specifically for older adults are delivered through the Older Americans Act. The OAA of 1965 was one of several major federal initiatives of President Lyndon B. Johnson's Great Society programs designed to benefit older persons (Estes, 1979). Today, the OAA has firmly established the aging network, including 57 State units on aging, approximately 650 Area Agencies on Aging, and 220 Tribal Organizations representing 300 Native Tribes (Takamura, 2001). While the mission of most ASOs is to serve persons living with or affected by HIV/AIDS, the aging network was designed specifically for older adults (typically defined as age 60). Acknowledging the aging population as an emerging group with growing social needs, the OAA developed to address those needs at the community level (Strupp, 2000).

In their analysis of these systems, Emlet and Poindexter (2004) demonstrate parallel structures between Ryan White funded program and those sponsored under the Older Americans Act. Both systems target specific populations; both must be reauthorized periodically; both are block grant programs originating with the federal Department of Health and Human Services and are delivered through state and local entities, which determine need and subcontract for service delivery; and both address the importance of consumer input and local decision making in the governance and allocation of resources. Under both systems, the core of services is provided to the target population at the local level. Both acts provide case management, counseling, and referrals, and both acts allow for services for family members and caregivers.

Despite the availability of programs throughout the United States at the local level, co-ordination between these systems has developed in only a relatively small number of geographic areas (see Nokes, 2004). Personnel from these systems do not typically communicate or attempt to coordinate services (Topolski, Gotham, Klinkenberg, O'Neill, & Brooks, 2002). Additionally, each service sector is characterized by philosophical or knowledge barriers that may prevent comprehensive and sensitive care to older adults living with HIV/AIDS. Joslin and Nazon (1996) suggest that the combination of ageism, homophobia, and AIDS-phobia among professionals in these systems contribute to creating barriers to care for this population.

As ASOs have primarily served younger persons, the needs of older adults have remained relatively invisible in that system (Joslin & Nazon, 1996). In a recent study of older Floridians with HIV/AIDS, Nichols and colleagues (2002) found some older clients hesitant to access HIV services due to the stigma attached to being older and HIV-positive. As HIV is not a disease typically associated with aging, social workers employed in the aging network may feel unfamiliar and uncomfortable with issues related to sexuality and HIV among older persons (Emlet & Poindexter, 2004). For example, Nichols and colleagues reported that older HIV consumers found seeking assistance from social services in general (not specifically from the aging network) to be uncomfortable and demeaning.

So while older adults with HIV/AIDS may access services developed through these two pieces of federal legislation, both systems and networks have their own barriers and perspectives that may encourage or deter use by older persons.

THEORETICAL BACKGROUND

This research was informed by the behavioral model of service utilization developed by Andersen (1968) and revised by Andersen and Newman (1973). This model has become a widely adopted conceptual framework for studying the use of health services (Wan, 1989; Wolinsky, 1988; Wolinsky, 1994) and has been successfully used in the analysis of data focusing on HIV/AIDS and service utilization (Hellinger, Fleishman, & Hsia, 1994; London, LeBlanc, & Aneshensel, 1998; Emlet, 1998).

The model suggests a sequence of conditions contribute to the volume of services used, including: (1) a predisposition of the individual to use services; (2) the ability to secure services; and (3) the need for such services (Andersen, 1968). The Predisposing Component is based on the premise that some individuals have a propensity to use services more than others. The Enabling Component of the model recognizes that even if an individual is predisposed to use health services, some means must be available for them to do so. The Need (or Illness Level) Component suggests that assuming the presence of predisposing and enabling conditions, an individual must perceive illness or the threat of illness to use health services.

METHODS

Participants and Procedures

The study was conducted in 2002/2003 in collaboration with an AIDS service organization (ASO) in the Pacific Northwest. This ASO is the primary ASO for the county and provides a variety of services including: case management, mental health and chemical dependency services, housing, and risk reduction/healthy behavior training. According to agency data, 12.3% of undup-
licated clients are age 50 and over, approximating the percentage of older adults living with HIV found in national statistics and in Washington State.

As part of the cooperative research agreement, case managers from the ASO contacted clients (both active and inactive) in the agency database who were 50 years of age or older, notifying them of the opportunity to participate in this study. Because of the relatively small number of individuals age 50 and over, purposive sampling techniques were used. During the initial contact (typically by phone), the study was briefly described; for those interested, an appointment was made for a face-to-face interview with the principal investigator or a research assistant. At that initial appointment, the study was described in detail, and participants who wished to continue signed the informed consent. Interviews lasted 45 minutes to one hour. All but one of the interviews was completed in English, with the exception conducted in Spanish through an interpreter. After the survey was successfully completed, participants were given $25 for their participation. The University's institutional review board (IRB) for the protection of human subjects approved all study procedures.

During the interview process, participants answered a series of questions related to socio-demographic characteristics. These items can be found in Table 1. Participants were then asked to review 10 types of services commonly provided to persons living with HIV/AIDS. This list represented a range of services from those associated with health promotion and wellness to public health programs (such as partner notification) and care and treatment (such as the AIDS drug assistance programs, clinical drug trials, case management services, and mental health counseling for persons living with HIV disease). Participants were asked to indicate if they had ever heard of or ever used these various programs or services. Data were collected dichotomously as a yes/no answer, so the amount or frequency of use was not assessed.

Participants were then asked to review a list of 10 services commonly available to older adults, and typically offered through the local area agency on aging or other local governmental or nonprofit agencies. The list of older adults services included: information and assistance programs, health promotion programs for older persons, senior centers, home and congregate meal programs, counseling services, assisted living facilities, adult day care programs, legal assistance and in-home chore services. Participants were asked if they had ever heard of these programs or services and if they had personally used them. The local availability of services from both networks were validated by personnel from the ASO and the area agency on aging. This research did not, however, incorporate standardized instruments into the design, thus no information on validity and reliability is provided.

RESULTS

Sample Characteristics

The analysis of sample characteristics is shown in Table 1. The 41 subjects in this analysis ranged in age from 50 to 71 years with a mean age of 55.66 years (SD 5.45). Ten of the 41 individuals (22.7%) were 60 years of age or over. The majority of respondents were male (70.7%). As shown in Table 1, approximately 68% were Caucasian with 22% African American. The remainder of subjects were Hispanic or other, which included individuals who self-identified as biracial. With regard to living arrangements, approximately half of these individuals lived alone; approximately 44% lived with a spouse, partner or other relative. The remaining 7% lived in other situations, such as clean-and-sober housing or shelters.

The educational level of the sample ranged from 7 to 17 years of education, with a mean of 13.17 years (SD = 2.34). Approximately 66 percent had no more than a high school education. Seven percent had a four year college degree or higher. Approximately half of the subjects were retired, with 22% being unemployed. Approximately one quarter worked part or full time. Although monthly income varied from under $400 to over $4,000, the majority of subjects were of low or moderate income. The poverty guidelines for 2003 place the poverty level for one individual at approximately $750 per month (Federal Register, 2003). Using these guidelines, 41.5% of the sample had individual incomes near or under the poverty level. Over 50 percent of the sample received Medicaid within 12 months prior to the interview.

Approximately 39 percent of the sample had been exposed to HIV through men having sex with men (MSM) or MSM combined with injection drug use. A similar proportion (44 percent) had been exposed through heterosexual sex. Slightly less than 10 percent identified injection drug use as the mode of HIV transmission. Seventy percent of the sample had met CDC criteria for an AIDS

TABLE 1. Sample Characteristics (N = 41)

Variable	Mean (SD)	n	%
Age	55.66 (5.45)		
Male		29	70.7
Race/Ethnicity			
White		28	68.3
African American		9	22.0
Hispanic		3	7.3
Other		1	2.4
Living Arrangements			
Lives Alone		20	48.8
Lives with Family or Partner		18	43.9
Other		3	7.3
Education	13.17 (2.34)		
High School or Less		27	65.9
Current Employment			
Unemployed		9	22.0
Retired		20	48.8
Works Part or Full-Time		11	26.8
Other		1	2.4
Income			
Less than $400/mo		4	9.8
$400 – 799		13	31.7
$800 – 1199		7	17.1
$1200+		17	41.4
Medicaid		21	51.2
HIV Exposure			
MSM		14	34.1
MSM/IVDU		2	4.9
Hetero		18	43.9
IVDU		4	9.8
Transfusion or Blood Products		1	2.4
Unknown		2	4.9
HIV/AIDS Status			
HIV		12	29.3
AIDS		29	70.7

diagnosis. These older respondents indicated a high degree of willingness to participate in the study. While some older individuals in the agency database could not be reached by phone or mail, of those older adults successfully contacted, 100% indicated a willingness to participate and successfully completed the interview.

Service Knowledge and Use

Knowledge of services from both systems is shown in Table 2. The majority of the respondents (N = 41) indicated knowledge of the existence of many of the HIV services listed, with the number of HIV related services ranging from 1 to 10 with a mean of 6.85 and a median of 8. Over 90 percent knew about case management and support group services. Nearly 80 percent were aware of HIV information hotlines. Over 70 percent knew of specialty mental health counseling and the availability of AIDS clinical drug trials, while sixty-three percent knew of the AIDS Drug Assistance Program. Fewer respondents were aware of HIV-related services such as partner notification typically provided through public health departments and health promotion and wellness programs.

The majority of respondents also were aware of many services provided through the aging network or of services designed primarily for older adults. Similar to the data seen in the HIV network, subjects indicated knowledge of an average of 6.15 aging services out of the 10 listed in the survey (the median was 3). As shown in Table 2, ninety percent of the participants were aware of home delivered meals, and over 80 percent were aware of assisted living facilities, in-home care or chore services and senior centers. While fewer in number, a majority (58.5%) had heard of adult day health care, and were aware of congregate meal sites (56.1%). The respondents were less familiar with senior information and assistance services, mental health counseling for older adults, and health promotion and wellness programs for older persons.

In relation to the use of HIV services, respondents used fewer services than they were aware of (6.85 in Table 2 versus 2.61 in Table 3). The most commonly used services from the HIV/AIDS system were case management and HIV support groups (87.8 and 43.9% respectively in Table 3). Additionally, a sizeable minority of older persons (nearly 32%) utilized the AIDS Drug Assistance Program as well as HIV-specific mental health counseling. Considerably fewer individuals utilized services such as HIV hotlines, partner notification, health promotion services, and legal assistance.

As seen in Table 3, the use of services differed across systems. Overall, respondents used lower levels of services in the aging network than the HIV network. While about 17 percent of these individuals used in-home care or chore services, use of most other aging network services ranged from two to ten percent. Approximately ten percent of the respondents had utilized senior centers, adult day programs, and home delivered meals. Slightly over seven percent had used Older American Act funded information and assistance programs and approximately five percent had used congregate senior meal sites.

The data were analyzed to determine if significant differences existed between knowledge and use within and across systems. This analysis is provided in Table 4. The means and medians from each service category (HIV awareness, HIV use, aging awareness and aging use) were compared using the

TABLE 2. Service Knowledge Among Older Adults with HIV/AIDS

Type of Service	Aware of Service n (%)
HIV/AIDS Services	
Case Management for PLWHIV	40 (97.6)
HIV Support Groups	39 (95.1)
HIV Information Hotline or Referral Line	32 (78.0)
HIV Specific Mental Health Counseling	30 (73.2)
AIDS Clinical Drug Trials	29 (70.7)
HIV/AIDS Housing Facilities	28 (68.3)
AIDS Drug Assistance Program	26 (63.4)
Legal Assistance for Persons with HIV/AIDS	25 (61.0)
Health Promotion and Wellness for HIV/AIDS	17 (41.5)
Partner Notification Program	16 (39.0)
Means/Median for HIV Services	6.85/8.00
Services for Older Adults	
Meals on Wheels	37 (90.2)
Assisted Living Facilities	34 (82.9)
In Home Care and Chore Programs	34 (82.9)
Senior Centers	33 (80.5)
Adult Day Health Care	24 (58.5)
Senior (Congregate) Meal Sites	23 (56.1)
Senior Information and Assistance Programs	18 (43.9)
Health Promotion and Wellness Programs for Older Adults	17 (41.5)
Legal Assistance of Older Adults	17 (41.5)
Mental Health Counseling for Older Adults	15 (36.6)
Means/Median for Senior Services	6.15/3.00

Wilcoxon Sign Test; a nonparametric test used in place of t-tests when one or more conditions for the use of parametric tests cannot be met (Weinbach & Grinnell, 2001). This form of analysis was chosen because of the strongly skewed distribution of counts which violate the assumptions of normality.

Table 4 reveals significant differences between knowledge and use of services within both systems as well as knowledge and use across systems. Individuals in this sample were significantly more likely to be aware of HIV services than to use them (Wilcoxon $Z = -6.41$; $p < .001$). The same holds true for services associated with the aging network (Wilcoxon $Z = -5.46$; $p < .001$). While the differences between awareness of services (HIV and aging) were statistically significant, overall differences in the medians were rela-

TABLE 3. Service Use Among Older Adults with HIV/AIDS

Type of Service	Use of Service n (%)
HIV/AIDS Services	
Case Management for PLWHIV	36 (87.8)
HIV Support Groups	18 (43.9)
HIV Specific Mental Health Counseling	16 (39.0)
AIDS Drug Assistance Program	13 (31.7)
AIDS clinical drug trials	9 (22.0)
Legal Assistance for Persons with HIV/AIDS	8 (19.5)
Health Promotion and Wellness for HIV/AIDS	4 (9.8)
HIV Information Hotline or Referral Line	2 (4.9)
Partner Notification Program	1 (2.4)
HIV/AIDS Housing Facilities	0 (0)
Means/Median for HIV Services	2.61/6.00
Services for Older Adults	
In Home care and chore programs	7 (17.1)
Meals on Wheels	4 (9.8)
Senior Centers	4 (9.8)
Adult Day Health Care	4 (9.8)
Senior Information and Assistance Programs	3 (7.3)
Senior (Congregate) Meal Sites	2 (4.9)
Assisted Living Facilities	1 (2.4)
Health Promotion and Wellness Programs for Older Adults	1 (2.4)
Legal Assistance of Older Adults	1 (2.4)
Mental Health Counseling for Older Adults	1 (2.4)
Means/Median for Senior Services	.68/0

tively small (8 compared to 6; Wilcoxon $Z = .041$; $p < .05$). The analytic elements in which differences were most notable were in the use of HIV versus aging services. While respondents used, on average, 2.61 HIV services (median = 3), the same individuals used an average of 0.68 aging services (median = 0) ($Z = -5.29$; $p < .001$).

Multivariate Analysis

To determine individual characteristics associated with knowledge and use of services from both systems, a logistic regression analysis was conducted guided by the Anderson framework. This framework acknowledges that indi-

TABLE 4. Comparative Analysis of Service Knowledge and Use

Service Comparison	Sig
HIV Services: Awareness and Use	$p < .001$
HIV and Aging Services: Awareness	$p < .05$
Aging Services Awareness and Use	$p < .001$
HIV and Aging Services: Use	$p < .001$

vidual attributes such as gender and ethnicity, access to services, and actual or perceived need may influence service use. Therefore, age, gender, ethnicity, Medicaid eligibility, and diagnosis (HIV versus AIDS) were used as independent variables in the model. The awareness of and use of both HIV and aging services were dichotomized using naturally occurring cut points in their distribution and placed in the model as dependant variables. As seen in Table 5, the only socio-demographic characteristic that emerged as significant when examining knowledge of HIV services was ethnicity. Individuals who were White had a 2.7 times greater likelihood of hearing of HIV services than their counterparts of color. To examine the use of services, we added, "having heard of the service" to the model.

The only independent variable significantly associated with use was having heard of the service. Those who had heard of the service were three times more likely to use the service than those that had not. With regard to aging services, the conceptual framework utilized showed poor predictability in terms of factors associated with hearing of aging services. None of the independent variables introduced into the model rose to the level of statistical significance at the .05 level. With regard to use of aging services, however, several important variables emerged as significant. As seen in Table 5, living arrangement, having received Medicaid in the past year and having heard of the service were predictive of using aging services while controlling for other variables in the model. Individuals who lived with others were 12.8 times less likely to use aging services than those who did not live with others, while having been enrolled in Medicaid increased one's likelihood of using aging services 15 times. Having heard of the service increased the likelihood of use over 18 times.

DISCUSSION

The purpose of this study was to examine the knowledge and use of services by older adults with HIV/AIDS. Two systems of service provision, those from the HIV network and those from the aging network, were explored. Overall, the data indicated moderate to high levels of knowledge of HIV services in this

TABLE 5. Significant Associations Based on Multivariate Logistic Regression[1]

Independent Variable	Heard of HIV Services		Use of HIV Services		Heard of Aging Services		Use of Aging Services	
	Odds Ratio	P	Odds Ratio	P	Odds Ratio	P	Odds Ratio	P
Age								
Gender								
Ethnicity	.36	.044						
Living With Others							.07	.045
Medicaid							15.58	.015
Heard of Service			3.47	.022			18.27	.053

[1]Significant associations are shown in the table. Non-significant associations are indicated by blank cells.

sample. Since the majority of subjects had been recruited from a local AIDS service organization, this should not be surprising. Those individuals who expressed a relatively high awareness of HIV services also used a number of important services from that system of care. Case management services, support groups for persons with HIV, mental health counseling, and the use of the AIDS Drug Assistance Program were among the most frequently used services. Having heard of the service was the only significant predictor of use when controlling for other factors. As knowledge of a service as a prerequisite to use appears obvious, it requires us to look at this picture with a broader lens. These data, for example, found that being White increased the likelihood of hearing about HIV services by 2.7 times and Whites were significantly more likely to have heard of a service than their counterparts of color. Having heard of the service then increased the likelihood of use more than three times. These findings suggest that HIV service providers need to increase outreach efforts to persons of color and older persons of color in particular.

While individuals in this study appeared to possess a similar level of awareness of services designed for older adults, they used far fewer aging services. Having Medicaid, hearing of the service and living with others were significant predictors of use. The services from the aging system that were most frequently used were in-home care and chore services. These were used at nearly twice the frequency of other services in that system. These findings parallel those of Emlet and Berghuis (2002), who found that among differences in service use among older versus younger individuals with HIV/AIDS, increased use among older persons appears to be associated with services which can be considered community-based long term care services designed primarily to help maintain one's independence. As receiving chore services is often dependent upon Medicaid eligibility, services from the aging network might be used only when perceived as necessary by the client (perhaps when functional dependency requires). While this study found the vast majority of older adults in this study did not turn to services administered through the aging network, the services that were used seemed to support independent functioning and did not duplicate services of the HIV network. In order for services to be used they must be available, accessible and acceptable (Wallace, 1990). Persons with HIV disease may simply feel more comfortable accessing help and assistance through the HIV network, particularly those whose lifestyles are perceived to be less acceptable to mainstream senior service providers. Thus, real or imagined stigma may play a role in where one seeks out services.

Do older persons with HIV/AIDS require and need access to both systems of care? In a recent article on service integration, Messeri, Kim, and Whetten (2003) provide a useful taxonomy for integration of HIV services, suggesting that the integration process can occur at client-centered, program-centered as well as policy-centered levels. Their model suggests that as long as needed services are accessed through a client-centered level of integration, this may be sufficient. At the same time, however, our findings suggest that knowledge of aging services is also a significant predictor of use. It is reasonable, therefore, for ASOs serving increasing numbers of older clients to move toward a beginning dialogue with older adult services in their communities. Such service integration activities can include case management services, case conferencing and written linkage agreement and do not necessarily involve large-scale administrative integration (Messeri et al., 2003). This type of communication has occurred in HIV epicenters with large numbers of older infected persons. An example of such communication and coordination can be found within the New York Association on HIV Over Fifty. The New York City HIV/AIDS and Aging Task Force was created in 1991 to bring professionals from AIDS and aging networks together to address the impact of the HIV/AIDS epidemic on older adults (Nokes, 2004). The association currently has approximately 80 members, including health and social service professionals, as well as older consumers who are living with HIV/AIDS. The association is an exemplar of a long-standing coalition operated under the model of shared governance (Nokes, 2004). Other geographical areas have also developed AIDS and aging task forces of various organizational types including Miami, New Jersey, Chicago, Boston and other cities (NAHOF, 2002). A listing of aging and HIV task forces can be found on the website for the National Association on HIV Over Fifty (NAHOF) at *www.hivoverfifty.org*.

Some important limitations existed within this study. First, subjects were obtained through purposive sampling techniques. These individuals were, therefore, self-selected, all recruited through the auspices of an AIDS Service Organization and consequently may have had higher levels of knowledge about HIV services than older adults not associated with an ASO. Additionally, purposive sampling itself produces some sampling bias. Another important limitation of this study was that data collection did not ascertain the amount of services used, only that a type of service had been used at some time.

According to recently released CDC data, nearly 61,000 persons age 50 and over were living with AIDS at the end of the year 2000 (CDC, 2003), figures do not account for older persons living with HIV. As the numbers of older adults living with HIV/AIDS continues to grow in the coming years, coordination of services between systems will take on increased importance. Additional research in this area can determine if the findings from this study hold true for larger, more generalizable populations of older persons and identify additional factors that facilitate or hinder the use of various services. The issues examined here will take on increasing importance in the coming years, requiring continuing examination of service utilization for this population.

REFERENCES

Andersen, R. (1968). *A behavioral model of families' use of health services*. Research Series No. 25. Chicago: Center for Health Administration Studies, University of Chicago.

Andersen, R., & Newman, J. F. (1973). Societal and individual determinants of medical care utilization in the United States. *Milbank Memorial Fund Quarterly, 51,* 95-124.

Center for Disease Control and Prevention [CDC] (2003). AIDS cases in adolescents and adults, by age–United States, 1994-2000. *HIV/AIDS Surveillance Supplemental Report, 9*(1), 1-25.

Crystal, S., LoSasso, A. T., & Sambamoorthi, U. (1999). Incidence and duration of hospitalizations among persons with AIDS: An event history approach. *Health Services Research, 33,* 1611-1638.

Crystal, S., & Sambamoorthi, U. (1998). Health care needs and service delivery for older persons with HIV/AIDS: Issues and research challenges. *Research on Aging, 20,* 739-759.

Emlet, C. A. (1993). Service utilization among older people with AIDS: Implications for case management. *Journal of Case Management, 2*(4), 119-124.

Emlet, C. A. (1998). *Correlates of service utilization among persons with HIV/AIDS: Does age make a difference?* Unpublished dissertation, Case Western Reserve University, Cleveland, Ohio. University Microfilms No. 9904009.

Emlet, C. A., & Berghuis, J. (2002). Service priorities, use and needs: Views of older and younger consumers living with HIV/AIDS. *Journal of Mental Health and Aging, 8*(4), 307-318.

Emlet, C., & Poindexter, C. (2004). The unserved, unseen, and unheard: Integrating programs for HIV-infected and affected elders. *Health and Social Work,* April/May.

Estes, C. L. (1979). *The aging enterprise.* San Francisco: Jossey-Bass.

Federal Register. (2003, February). *68*(26), 6456-6458.

Fritsch, T. (2001). *HIV/AIDS and the older adults: An exploratory study of the age-related differences in access to medical and social services.* Unpublished master's thesis, Simon Fraser University, Vancouver, British Columbia, Canada.

Harel, Z., Noelker, L., & Blake, B. F. (1985). Comprehensive services for the aged: Theoretical and empirical perspectives. *The Gerontologist, 25,* 644-649.

Hellinger, F. J., Fleishman, J. A. & Hsia, D. C. (1994). AIDS treatment costs during the last months of life: Evidence from the ACSUS. *Health Services Research, 29,* 569-581.

Joslin, D., & Nazon, M. (1996). HIV/AIDS and aging networks. In. K. Nokes (Ed.). *HIV/AIDS and the older adult* (pp. 129-141). Bristol, PA: Taylor and Francis.

London, A. S., LeBlanc, A. J., & Aneshensel, C. S. (1998). The integration of informal care, case management and community-based services for persons with HIV/AIDS. *AIDS Care, 10*(4), 481-503.

Messeri, P., Kim, S., & Whetten, K. (2003). Measuring HIV services integration activities. *Journal of HIV/AIDS & Social Services, 2*(1), 19-44.

National Association on HIV Over Fifty [NAHOF] (2002, May). Resource Information: HIV Over Fifty. Retrieved April 16, 2003, from: http://www.hivoverfifty.org/nahof_resources.html

Nichols, J. E., Speer, D. C., Watson, B. J., Watson, M. R., Vergon, T. L., Valee, C. M. et al. (2002). *Aging with HIV: Psychological, social and health issues.* San Diego: Academic Press.

Nokes, K. (2004). *Sustaining a coalition: New York Association on HIV Over Fifty*. In C. A. Emlet (Ed.). *HIV/AIDS and older adults: Challenges for individuals, families and communities*. New York: Springer.

Strupp, H. W. (2000). Area Agencies on Aging: A national network of services to maintain elderly in their communities. *Care Management Journals, 2*(1), 54-62.

Takamura, J. C. (2001). Older Americans Act. In M. D. Mezey (ed.). *The Encyclopedia of elder care: The comprehensive resource on geriatric and social care* (pp. 468-471). New York: Springer.

Topolski, J. M., Gotham, H. J., Klinkenberg, W. D., O'Neill, D. L, & Brooks, A. R. (2002). Older adults, substance use and HIV/AIDS: Preparing for a future crisis. *Journal of Mental Health and Aging, 8*(4), 349-363.

Turner, B., Kelly, J. V., & Ball, J. K. (1989). A severity classification system for AIDS hospitalizations. *Medical Care, 27*, 423-437.

Turner, B. J., McKee, L., Fanning, T., & Markson, L. E. (1994). AIDS specialist versus generalist ambulatory care for advanced HIV infection and impact on hospital use. *Medical Care, 32*(9), 902-916.

Wallace, S. P. (1990). The no-care zone: Availability, accessibility, and acceptability in community-based long-term care. *The Gerontologist, 30*, 254-261.

Wan, T. T. H. (1989). The behavioral model of health care utilization by older people. In M. G. Ory and K. Bond (Eds.), *Aging and health care: Social science and policy perspectives* (pp. 52-77). New York: Routledge.

Weinbach, R. W., & Grinnel, R. M. (2001). *Statistics for social workers* (5th ed.). Needham Heights, MA: Allyn and Bacon.

Wolinsky, F. D. (1988). The sociology of health: Principles, practitioners and issues. Belmont, CA: Wadsworth.

Wolinsky, F. D. (1994). Health service utilization by older adults: Conceptual, measurement and modeling issues in secondary analysis. *The Gerontologist, 34*, 470-475.

Perceptions of Vulnerability to HIV Among Older African American Women: The Role of Intimate Partners

April Winningham, DrPH
Donna Richter, EdD
Sara Corwin, PhD
Cheryl Gore-Felton, PhD

SUMMARY. This is one of the first studies among older African American women to examine partner communication and perceived risk for

April Winningham, DrPH, is an NRSA Postdoctoral Fellow and Cheryl Gore-Felton, PhD, is Assistant Professor, both at the Medical College of Wisconsin, Department of Psychiatry & Behavioral Medicine, Center for AIDS Intervention Research.

Sara Corwin, PhD, is Research Assistant Professor and Donna Richter, PhD, is Interim Dean and Associate Dean for Public Health Practice at the University of South Carolina, Arnold School of Public Health.

Address correspondence to: Dr. Winningham, Medical College of Wisconsin, Center for AIDS Intervention Research (CAIR), 2071 North Summit Avenue, Milwaukee, WI 53202 (E-mail: awinning@mcw.edu).

The authors wish to acknowledge the contributions to this research by the American Cancer Society/Best Chance Network of South Carolina, Joyce Hudson, Pastor Betty Smith, Denyse Petry, Jane P. Fowler, Kathy Nokes, PhD, RN, FAAN, Cynthia Graham, PhD, Stephanie Sanders, PhD, William Yarber, HSD, and the women who participated in this study.

Preparation of this manuscript was supported, in part, by National Institute of Mental Health (NIMH) Center grant P30-MH52776 and National Research Service Award postdoctoral training grant T32-MH19985.

[Haworth co-indexing entry note]: "Perceptions of Vulnerability to HIV Among Older African American Women: The Role of Intimate Partners." Winningham, April et al. Co-published simultaneously in *Journal of HIV/AIDS & Social Services* (The Haworth Press) Vol. 3, No. , 2004, pp. 25-42; and: *Midlife and Older Adults and HIV: Implications for Social Service Research, Practice, and Policy* (ed: Cynthia Cannon Poindexter, and Sharon M. Keigher) The Haworth Press, Inc., 2004, pp. 25-42. Single or multiple copies of this article are available for a fee from The Haworth Document Delivery Service [1-800-HAWORTH, 9:00 a.m. - 5:00 p.m. (EST). E-mail address: docdelivery@haworthpress.com].

http://www.haworthpress.com/web/JHASO
Digital Object Identifier: 10.1300/J187v03n01_04

HIV. Understanding that the vast majority of older women are infected through heterosexual contact, this study investigated several partner-related factors associated with perceptions of vulnerability to HIV among older African American women (age range = 50-81 years). A cross-sectional survey was conducted (n = 167) in three rural counties in South Carolina. Perceptions of vulnerability to HIV was most strongly associated with women who were not married, believed that their sexual partner would not approve of using condoms and had more comfort in communicating with their partners about sex. Recognizing the role of intimate partners in predicting women's perceptions of their own vulnerability to HIV is an important factor to consider when developing HIV prevention programs for older African American women. Future studies need to examine factors associated with effective partner communication, particularly negotiation strategies around condom use among older adults. *[Article copies available for a fee from The Haworth Document Delivery Service: 1-800-HAWORTH. E-mail address: <docdelivery@haworthpress.com> Website: <http://www.HaworthPress.com> © 2004 by The Haworth Press, Inc. All rights reserved.]*

KEYWORDS. HIV/AIDS and women, rural, older adults, sexuality, perceived susceptibility, perceived vulnerability

The incidence of HIV is increasing among older women at such a fast rate that between 2000 and 2001 the number of HIV infections among older women increased by 51% (CDC, 2001; CDC, 2002). Despite the need for HIV prevention efforts among older women, particularly African American women living in rural southern communities, there is a paucity of research related to sexuality, HIV risk and prevention among this population. Although there are compelling psychosocial models of risk behavior that have been successfully applied to young African American women (Bachanas et al., 2002), few factors associated with risk behavior have been examined among older African American women. Understanding these factors will assist prevention efforts in developing effective methods to reduce the rising incidence of HIV among older women, especially those living in the southern region of the U.S. where the epidemic has hit the hardest. Based on the conceptual framework of the Health Belief Model, the purpose of this study is to explore factors associated with perceptions of vulnerability to HIV, a key component to behavior change, among older African American women living in rural South Carolina.

NEED FOR HIV PREVENTION
AMONG OLDER AFRICAN AMERICAN WOMEN

In the United States, the incidence of HIV infection and AIDS diagnosis is increasing most rapidly among African American women (Crosby, Yarber, DiClemente, Wingood, & Meyerson, 2002). Research indicates that of all newly reported AIDS cases in 1998, more women were in the South (41%), African American (61%), and infected by heterosexual transmission (38%) (Hader, Smith, Moore, & Holmberg, 2001). In 1999, HIV/AIDS was the third leading cause of death among African American women between the ages of 25 and 44 (CDC, 2000). Like their younger counterparts, older African American women (age 50 and older) are also disproportionately affected by the HIV/AIDS epidemic. African American women account for approximately 11% of all older women in the U.S. (United States Census Bureau, 2001) but account for more than 50% of AIDS cases among older women and more than 65% of HIV infections among older women (CDC, 2002). These percentages are even higher in some states like South Carolina where 78% of the women age 50 and older living with HIV are African American (South Carolina Department of Health and Environmental Control, 2001). Such trends indicate an ever-growing need to address HIV prevention among older African American women living in the South.

FACTORS ASSOCIATED WITH HIV/AIDS RISK BEHAVIORS
AMONG OLDER AFRICAN AMERICAN WOMEN

The disparity of HIV rates among older African American women living in the South may be due to the combination of their unique set of circumstances including: (1) physiological changes related to age; (2) living in the South, (3) living in rural areas, (4) lack of sexual negotiation skills, and (5) lack of perceived vulnerability to HIV.

Physiological Changes Related to Age. The normal aging process includes a decline in the immune system's ability to function properly (Moore & Amburgey, 2000). As a result, older adults may be at greater risk when exposed to HIV (Riley, 1997). Older women may be at additional risk for HIV infection during intercourse due to normal aging changes such as decreased vaginal lubrication and estrogen deficiencies which cause thinning of the vaginal walls (Moore & Amburgey, 2000; Whipple & Scura, 1996). These physiological changes allow for more tearing of the vaginal walls during sexual intercourse and provide a direct route for HIV transmission. Older women, then, are considered at greater risk for HIV transmission during sexual intercourse than younger women.

Living in the South. In 1999, CDC reported the highest AIDS rates among metropolitan areas. Three of the top four cities were located in the South–Ft.

Lauderdale, FL; Miami, FL; and Columbia, SC (Winiarski, 2000). In terms of regions of the U.S., a higher number of older adult HIV cases were reported in the Southern region in 2001 than in any other region of the country (CDC, 2001).

Living in Rural Areas. For those women living in South Carolina, a predominantly rural state, there are additional concerns and circumstances affecting rates of HIV/AIDS. The number of new AIDS cases is growing at an alarming rate in rural southern communities, especially among African Americans and those infected with HIV through heterosexual contact (DeCarlo, 1997). The rate of AIDS cases in rural areas rose 37% from 1991 to 1995, compared to only a 5% increase in metropolitan areas during that same time frame (Rural Center for the Study and Promotion of HIV/STD Prevention, 1996). Some studies have indicated that this increase in AIDS cases in rural areas has disproportionately affected African American women, with one study in rural Alabama indicating a 170-fold increase in AIDS cases among African American women over a 10-year period (Holmes et al., 1997). Further evidence (Crosby et al., 2002) indicates significantly more HIV-risk factors among rural African American women than among non-rural African American women. These risk factors included not using condoms, no HIV testing of sexual partner(s), no preferred method of prevention, a belief that their partner was HIV negative despite the lack of testing, and a lack of perceived vulnerability for HIV.

An additional burden often prevalent in rural communities is the lack of public health resources necessary to adequately address the HIV/AIDS epidemic. The lack of and inability to obtain public health resources is perpetuated by the common perception that HIV is not a problem in rural areas (Voelker, 1998).

Lack of Sexual Negotiation Skills. It is estimated that one in 50 African American men is infected with HIV (CDC, 2001). For African American women, including older women, having sexual contact with these men, there is an increased risk of heterosexually acquired HIV. Although condom usage may reduce their risk for HIV, African American women may not want to or may not be able to negotiate condom use. Inability or unwillingness to negotiate condom use may be due to beliefs that negotiating condoms would interfere with physical and emotional intimacy, imply infidelity by themselves or their partner, or result in physical abuse (Peterson et al., 1999).

In focus group research conducted with African American women between the ages of 18 and 44, the following reasons were offered for unprotected sexual activity: "negative attitudes toward condoms, refusal by men to use condoms, refusal by women to negotiate condom use, and the belief that 'some people just don't care [about protecting themselves]'" (Timmons & Sowell, 1999, p. 585). St. Lawrence, Eldridge, Reitman, Little, Shelby and Brasfield (1998) theorize that "condoms also are viewed negatively within the African American community because of their association with casual relationships, infidelity, disease, and because of beliefs that they detract from trust, intimacy and commitment in a relationship" (p. 9).

Perceived Vulnerability. In 1998, the Congressional Black Caucus declared a state of emergency in the African American community due to the devastating consequences of the AIDS epidemic (Cornelius, Okundaye, & Manning, 2000). Despite that declaration, many African American communities still view HIV/AIDS primarily as a gay issue (Cornelius et al., 2000). Due to the prevalence of this misperception, women within these communities may be unaware or in denial of their own risk for HIV infection (Peterson, Wingood, DiClemente, DeCarlo, & Quirk, 1999). Very little is known about perceived vulnerability to HIV among older adults. However, a national survey study conducted by the Centers for Disease Control and Prevention (CDC; Ory & Mack, 1998) suggests that adults age 50 and older perceive themselves to be at low risk for HIV. Some have speculated that older adults do not use condoms because they may not feel susceptible to sexually transmitted infections (STIs), such as HIV, and because they may no longer have a need for birth control (Nokes, 1996; Whipple & Scura, 1996). Indeed, due to a lack of perceived vulnerability to HIV, older adults may be more likely to engage in sexual behaviors that put them at risk for HIV. Therefore, understanding factors associated with perceived vulnerability among older adults, particularly those that are most at risk for HIV, is an important first step in prevention efforts.

USING THEORY TO ASSIST IN UNDERSTANDING RISK BEHAVIOR

Behavioral theories allow us to explain and predict behavior. Without theories or models, it would be almost impossible to develop an intervention or prevention program because we wouldn't know what behaviors, thoughts, or even emotions were important to intervene on to get our desired outcome of reduced risk. For more than thirty years, one of the most widely used theories to explain health-related behavior is the Health Belief Model (HBM; Hochbaum, 1958; Rosenstock, 1960, 1966, 1974). According to HBM, before an individual makes a commitment to changing behavior, the individual must first perceive themselves as being susceptible or vulnerable to a health threat, such as HIV. Understanding factors associated with perceived vulnerability or perceived risk of getting HIV is important because findings such as these can provide a scientific rationale for intervention strategies, thereby improving the likelihood that strategies will be effective. Indeed, prevention studies among African American adults based upon principles of the HBM have been effective in reducing risk behavior (DiClemente & Wingood, 1995; Wingood & DiClemente, 1996; Wingood & DiClemente, 1998). Because HIV transmission occurs within couple relationships, the traditional models of health-related behavior need to take into account behaviors, cognitions, and emotions associated with intimate partner relationships. For women, this is particularly important, given that the primary route of HIV transmission is through heterosexual contact. Thus, it is essential to consider sexual partners in models that examine women's perceived vulnerability to HIV.

Few studies have been conducted that examine perceptions of HIV risk among older women. Moreover, to our knowledge, there are no studies that have examined risk perceptions of older African American women living in the South. Understanding risk perceptions is an important first step in developing prevention messages, intervention programs, and services for women who are at increasing risk for HIV infection. Therefore, we examined factors associated with perceived vulnerability to HIV among older African American women living in rural South Carolina.

METHODS

Study Participants. The sample demographics are shown in Table 1. Nearly half of the women (48%) had less than a high school education with 12% having never attended school. Most women (58%) were not married, nor living with a partner.

Sampling Design. This descriptive study utilized a cross-sectional survey design with a convenience sample of participants. Individuals who met the selection criteria of gender (female), age (age 50 and older), race (African American), and county of residence (3 rural counties selected for the study) were recruited to complete a paper-and-pencil survey instrument that had been pilot tested. Approval to conduct the study was obtained from the sponsoring research institution's human subjects review board.

Sample Recruitment. This study was conducted with the assistance of staff from an ongoing breast cancer screening program known as the Best Chance Network (BCN). Associating HIV with other preventable health behaviors was an effective way to gain access to older African American women living in rural counties. The BCN provides free cancer screenings to women who are: (1) between the ages of 47 and 64, (2) do not have health insurance, or have health insurance which only pays for hospital care, and (3) meet annual family income guidelines. Annual income guidelines range from $15,244 or less for a family of one to $36,112 for a family of five. From February 1-March 31, 2002, two female outreach liaisons from BCN recruited 209 women from communities in three selected rural counties for this study. Once informed consent was obtained, participants were scheduled to complete the survey.

Data Collection. Two trained female interviewers administered the survey. To increase participation rates and reduce potential transportation barriers, the paper-and-pencil questionnaires were administered in small groups in community churches or in participants' homes. To increase reading comprehension and to allow women with lower literacy skills to fully participate, each

TABLE 1. Descriptive Statistics of Sample Demographics (n = 167)

Variable	%
Age	
50-54	37.7
55-59	22.8
60-64	26.9
65-69	9.0
70-74	2.4
75-81	1.2
Marital Status	
Married/Living with Partner	42.5
Separated	11.4
Divorced	22.8
Widowed	17.4
Never Married	6.0
Education	
Never Attended School	12.0
Grades 1-8	19.2
Grades 9-11	16.8
Grade 12 or GED	31.1
College 1-3 years	14.4
College 4+ years	6.6

Note: Percentages may not equal 100% due to the rounding of decimal places.

question and corresponding response options were read aloud by trained staff to each small group of participants. The questionnaires required 45-55 minutes to complete and were sealed in individual, unmarked manila envelopes by each participant upon completion.

Of the 209 collected surveys, forty-two were excluded from the analyses because of a failure to meet one or more of the study's inclusion criteria of race (African American, n = 7), age (50 years of age or older, n = 4), or county of residence (one of three designated rural counties, n = 12) or were excluded because of significant missing data (n = 19). A total of 167 women were included in the data analysis.

Study Measures. Measures for this study include demographics, partner approval of condom usage, partner-risk behaviors, self-risk behaviors, comfort with partner communication, response efficacy, and perceived vulnerability.

Demographics. Demographic factors included county of residence, age, marital/partner status and education level.

Partner Approval. Partner approval was assessed with a single-item measure utilized previously with African American women (St. Lawrence et al., 1998), "If you were in a sexual relationship with a male sexual partner, how much would he approve of using a condom?" Responses ranged from (1) = "strongly agree" to (5) = "strongly disagree" on a Likert-type response scale. Scores were reversed so that a higher score indicated greater partner approval of condom use.

Partner-Risk Behaviors. Adapted from previous studies with women (Gielen et al., 1994), HIV-related risk behaviors of sexual partners within the last five years were assessed with 5 items: (1) partner having had a blood transfusion between 1978 and 1985, (2) partner infected with HIV, (3) partner having injected heroin, speed or cocaine, (4) partner also having sex with other women, and (5) partner also having sex with other men. Prior to the pilot test of the survey instrument, women were presented with two responses to these questions: yes or no. During the pilot testing phase of this study, women recommended including "I don't know" as a response to partner behaviors in order to allow women to "air" their suspicions without making accusations in writing. Therefore, we added "I don't know" to the survey responses. For the purposes of this study's analyses, we scored "yes" and "I don't know" responses as 1 and "no" as 0. Coding the data in this way confers risk on absolute assertions as well as unknown responses. This strategy is consistent with CDC prevention messages that encourage individuals to get tested for HIV if they are having sex with someone who is either known to be HIV infected or has an unknown serostatus. According to the CDC, those having sex with a partner with an unknown serostatus are considered at risk for infection. The CDC took this conservative stance because it is estimated that 25% of the people living with HIV don't know that they are infected (CDC, 2003), which poses a serious public health threat. Responses were summed across all items for a total score, which created a partner-risk behavior index ranging from 0 to 5.

Self-Risk Behaviors. Adapted from previous studies with women (Binson, Pollack, & Catania, 1997; Gielen et al., 1994), HIV-related risk behaviors during the past five years were assessed with four items: (1) history of multiple (i.e., 2 or more) sex partners, (2) history of exchanging sex for something of value (i.e., money or drugs), (3) history of injecting heroin, speed, or cocaine, and (4) history of practicing anal sex. Affirmative responses were given a score of 1 and negative responses scored 0. The scores were summed to create the self-risk behavior index ranging from 0 to 4.

Comfort with Partner Communication. Partner communication was assessed with a 3-item scale adapted from previous research with African American women (St. Lawrence et al., 1998). Ratings were on a 1 to 5 Likert-type response scale ranging from "very uncomfortable" to "completely comfortable." Responses to items such as, "If you wanted to discuss using a condom with a sexual partner, how would you feel?" were summed to create a total score. Higher scores indicate a greater level of comfort in communicating with a partner about sex. Cronbach's alpha indicated that the internal consistency of the scale was .73.

Response Efficacy. Response efficacy, or the belief that condoms are effective against HIV transmission, was a single-item measure previously utilized with women (Kline & VanLandingham, 1994), "I believe that condoms are very helpful in protecting a person from getting HIV." Responses ranged from (1) = "strongly agree" to (5) = "strongly disagree" on a Likert-type response scale. Scores were reversed so that a higher score indicated a greater belief that condoms were effective in protecting against HIV transmission.

Perceived Vulnerability. Utilized previously with women, the perceived vulnerability scale (Gielen, Faden, O'Campo, Kass, & Anderson, 1994) is a self-report measure of an individual's perceived vulnerability to HIV infection. The original scale is composed of five items; however, in this study, the following two items were omitted: "Given my lifestyle, there is a chance I could get AIDS" and "I'm afraid I could get AIDS from a sexual partner." Internal consistency reliability estimates using Cronbach's alpha increased from .25 to .75 once these items were removed. Therefore, only the first three items were used to determine participants' perceived vulnerability to HIV, which included, "I can't get AIDS because my sexual partner(s) has (have) been very clean." Responses ranged from "strongly agree" to "strongly disagree" on a 5 point Likert-type response scale. The mean scale score was calculated by summing the responses and dividing by the number of items. A higher scale score indicated a stronger perception of vulnerability to HIV.

Data Analyses. Completed surveys were manually reviewed, coded and prepared for entry into EPI INFO (v. 6.04b). To minimize data entry errors, the surveys were entered twice with data files cross-validated. Any errors found during this process were corrected. After the data were entered and validated, the file was exported from EPI INFO (v. 6.04b) into SAS (Stokes, Davis, & Koch, 1995) for further data analysis.

To examine the association of perceived vulnerability to HIV with demographic variables, partner approval of using condoms, partner behavior risk, comfort with partner communication, and response efficacy, we conducted a hierarchical linear multiple regression with perceived vulnerability as the dependent variable. A linear regression is a mathematical technique used to fit variables to a straight line to predict an outcome, which in this study was perceived vulnerability. In hierarchical regressions, the researcher decides which variables to put into the equation in a specific order. The order is guided by standard practices within a field of study as well as theoretical considerations. In this study, to control for the possible influence of residence on perceived vulnerability, we entered county of residence into the first block. It is standard practice when conducting a study at different sites to control for any site differences that might occur. These differences might be due to chance, an unforeseen event (e.g., a county health fair) or some other unknown factor. Because it is not possible to detail all the reasons a particular site might differ from another, the effects of any site differences must be controlled in the regression analyses. Demographic variables (age, marital status, and education level) were placed into the second block using the stepwise forward procedure. In the third and final block, the remaining variables of interest: partner approval, partner-risk, partner communication and efficacy were simultaneously entered. To control for multicollinearity, self-risk was not included in the model because of its strong association with partner-risk (r = 0.60, p < .001).

RESULTS

Almost one-quarter (24%) of the sample reported being married/partnered with at least one partner-risk behavior and 20% reported being married/partnered with at least one self-risk behavior. Moreover, more than one-quarter (26%) of the sample who reported a partner-risk also reported a lower perception of vulnerability to HIV. Among women who reported at least one self-risk behavior or at least one partner-risk behavior, 32% also reported lower perceptions of vulnerability to HIV. Women who reported self-risk behavior were significantly more likely to report a lowered perception of vulnerability to HIV compared to those who did not report self-risk (t = −3.85, p < .001).

More than half of the women (59%) were categorized as having a partner who had engaged in at least one of five HIV risk-related behaviors. Of those women (n = 99), the partner's risk ranged from also having sex with other women (77%), also having sex with men (33%), injecting drugs (36%), having a blood transfusion between 1978 and 1985 (41%), and being infected with HIV (29%).

Nearly half (46%) of the women reported at least one of the four self-risk behaviors, with nearly one-quarter (23%) reporting two or more self-risk behaviors. Of those reporting at least one self-risk behavior (n = 77), more than two-thirds (69%) reported multiple partners, about half (51%) reported participating in anal sex, and almost one-third reported injecting drugs (30%) and exchanging sex for something of value (29%). Overall, more than one-third of the sample (40%) reported at least one self-risk behavior and at least one partner-risk behavior.

Descriptive statistics of the variables of interest are shown in Table 2. A median split on the perceived vulnerability scores indicated that 50% of the women reported low perceived risk and 50% reported high risk. The average scores of perceived vulnerability (mean = 2.9) and comfort with partner communication (mean = 9.2) fell in the middle of the score ranges. On average, the number of reported partner risks for this population was 1.3 out of a range of 0-5 risks. The average scores for partner approval for condom usage (mean = 3.7) and response efficacy or the belief in the effectiveness of condoms (mean = 4.0) were closer to the high end of the scales rather than the lower end.

TABLE 2. Descriptive Statistics of Variables of Interest (n = 167)

Study Variables	Mean	SD	Range
Perceived Vulnerability	2.9	1.1	1-5
Scores range from low perception of vulnerability (1) to high perception of vulnerability (5)			
Partner-Risk	1.3	1.4	0-5
Scores range from no partner risks (0) to high number of partner risk behaviors (5)			
Partner Approval for Condom Usage	3.7	1.4	1-5
Scores range from low approval (1) to high approval (5)			
Comfort with Partner Communication	9.2	4.1	3-15
Scores range from low levels of comfort (3) to high levels of comfort (15)			
Response Efficacy: Belief that condoms are effective	4.0	1.1	1-5
Scores range from low belief in condom effectiveness (1) to high belief in condom effectiveness (5)			

As seen in Table 3, the overall regression model to predict perceptions of vulnerability to HIV was statistically significant ($F[7,159] = 10.045$, $p < .001$), and resulted in an adjusted $R^2 = .28$, indicating that the model accounted for nearly 30% of the variance in perceived vulnerability. In other words, the results of this analysis indicated that partner-related factors (marital status, partner approval to use condoms, partner's risk behaviors, comfort with partner communication and response efficacy) accounted for a significant amount of the variability in women's perceptions of their own vulnerability to HIV. Older women who were single, did not believe that their partner would approve of using condoms, and were comfortable in communicating with their partner about sex were more likely to feel more vulnerability to HIV.

As illustrated in Table 3, the (Beta) coefficient shown in the second column indicates the relative magnitude and the direction of the relationship of each independent variable to the dependent variable. Women who were not married or living with a partner reported greater perceptions of vulnerability to HIV compared to those who were married/partnered. Greater partner approval for using condoms was significantly associated with lower perceived vulnerability to HIV. Interestingly, women who reported greater comfort with partner communication were significantly more likely to report greater perceived vulnerability for HIV.

DISCUSSION

Many of the women in this study are single and may find themselves looking for a partner in the era of HIV, without an awareness of the risks to them-

TABLE 3. Summary of Hierarchical Regression Analysis for Variables Predicting Women's Perceived Vulnerability to HIV

Independent Variable	SE B	β	t
County 1	0.17	0.07	1.00
County 2	0.28	−0.10	−1.34
Marital Status	0.15	−0.15	−2.21*
Partner Approval	0.06	−0.23	−3.18**
Partner-risk	0.06	0.01	0.14
Partner Communication	0.02	0.38	5.43***
Response Efficacy	0.07	−0.09	−1.29

Note: n = 167; full model adjusted R^2 = .28; $F(7,159)$ = 10.045, p < .001. The t values and β values are presented for the final regression model. Demographic variables that were not statistically significant in the second block using the stepwise forward procedure were dropped from the final regression model and therefore are not shown in the table.
*p < 0.04 **p < 0.005 ***p < 0.001

selves of engaging in unprotected sexual intercourse. This is evidenced by our findings that most women were not married and more than one-third of the women in the study reported self and partner behavior that put them at increased risk for HIV infection. Furthermore, approximately one-third of the sample reported low perceived risk in spite of reporting either self or partner-risk behavior. This is consistent with previous research in which rural African American women, compared to their non-rural counterparts, had significantly more HIV-risk factors including: not using condoms, no HIV testing of sexual partner(s), no preferred method of prevention, a belief that their partner was HIV negative, despite the lack of testing, and a lack of perceived vulnerability for HIV (Crosby et al., 2002). Moreover, a study among African American women found that when women felt safe in their intimate sexual relationships they did not use condoms (Timmons & Sowell, 1999).

Despite reporting personal and partner-related risk behaviors for HIV, half of the women in this study reported low perceptions of vulnerability to HIV. According to the Health Belief Model, in order to begin changing behavior, an individual must first acknowledge vulnerability to a health threat, such as HIV. Clearly, prevention efforts for this population must include in their initial focus the awareness that HIV transmission is based on *not who you are, but what you do.* This lack of perceived vulnerability to HIV among older African American women may also be prevalent among social workers, health educators and other social and health care professionals that are providing services to these women. Education and awareness of older adult HIV risk behaviors must be emphasized among all social service and health care providers when developing community-level HIV prevention efforts. Once aware, providers will reinforce the vulnerability of this population to HIV by inquiring about risk behaviors among older clients. Additional training for providers may be necessary in order to enhance their own comfort level in speaking with older clients about issues of sexuality and risk behaviors.

Findings of this study also have implications in terms of the prevention skills necessary for older African American women to protect themselves against HIV infection. Despite coming from an era where condom usage may not have been popular, many of the women reported that they believed that condoms were effective in preventing the spread of HIV and that their partners would approve of using condoms. Although social marketing and basic HIV education have not typically targeted this generation, this study's findings indicate that the message of condom effectiveness has reached members of this population. Transforming this perception of condom effectiveness into safer sex practice may be further assisted as many women in this study had strong beliefs that their partners would approve of using condoms. This provides a tremendous reinforcing platform upon which to build such prevention skills as condom negotiation and proper condom usage.

Also based on findings from this study, there are several cultural issues that must be further explored and addressed in order to provide comprehensive, effective HIV prevention efforts among this population. Based on self-reported risk behaviors, HIV prevention efforts among older African American women must also address risk behaviors of injection drug use (IDU) and higher risk behaviors such as anal sex and exchanging sex for something of value. Additionally, among the women who reported having a partner with at least one risk behavior, more than three-quarters had a sexual partner that was also having sex with other women. Future studies, particularly qualitative studies, must be conducted in order to better understand the context of these activities.

Low socioeconomic status of older African American women living in the South may play a role in choice of partner and perhaps the risk behavior of exchanging sex for something of value. Across all public health issues, economic status has often been linked directly and indirectly to behaviors. Airhihenbuwa, DiClemente, Wingood, and Lowe (1992) found that, like most Americans, "the daily behavioral choices of many African Americans are highly influenced by their economic situation" (p. 269). Lee, Ganges, Cross, and Garner (1999) emphasize that "because African Americans . . . suffer more from poverty, discrimination, a lack of access to health care and a lack of health insurance, they are at an increased risk for HIV and other infectious diseases" (p. 1).

Even more of a culturally taboo subject within the African American community is the issue of being on the "down low." This term, popularized in the media, refers to African American men who have sex with men but do not typically disclose this fact to female partners nor identify themselves as being gay (Sternberg, 2001). In this study, one-third of the women reported that they knew or were unsure if their partner was also having sex with men. Since the highest rates of HIV transmission are still among MSM, risk implications for women who are participating in sexual risk behaviors with men on the "down low" are enormous.

Much of what we know about risk behaviors, dating and sexual relationships comes from individuals between the ages of 18 and 44. We cannot assume that models that apply to young adults will also apply to older adults. For example, in this study we found that greater partner communication was associated with greater perceived vulnerability. This is counter to findings among young women by DiClemente and Wingood (1995) and St. Lawrence et al. (1998), where greater communication was associated with lower risk behavior and lower perceived risk, respectively. We believe one explanation for this difference may be contextual in that younger adults, particularly heterosexuals, are often in serial monogamous relationships. In addition, older adult women frequently return to dating after many years of being in a monogamous marriage/relationship that has ended due to death, divorce, or separation. Thus, the content of the sexual communication may be very different between these age cohorts by virtue of the different context in which the sexual relationship occurs. Also, older adults grew up in a time when there were many more social constraints on sexual behavior, particularly for women. So, sexual communication among older women with partners may be devoid of specific sexual behavior and/or needs. Clearly, more research is needed in this area to understand the mediating and moderating effects of communication on risk behavior among older women.

It is also important to note that, in our sample, a significant proportion of women had less than a high school education. Literacy, particularly health literacy, is an important factor in how individuals access and seek treatment and care. As we enter the next decade of HIV research and prevention, delivering prevention messages that are age-appropriate, clear and effective, is the challenge for health providers, public health officials, and researchers. This is especially challenging when the messages have to reach populations that do not believe themselves to be at risk for HIV and therefore, do not attend to the messages or seek prevention services.

This is one of the first studies among older African American women to examine partner communication and perceived risk for HIV. However, consistent with the observation of previous researchers (Catania et al., 1989), we still do not know how well older adults are able to negotiate changes in sexual behavior with their partners. Future studies need to examine factors associated with effective partner communication, particularly negotiation strategies around condom use among older adults.

In terms of implications for social workers and other social service providers, this study provides insights into practice, service and policy changes necessary to meet the needs of older African American women at risk for HIV. As this study indicates, older women and their sexual partners participate in activities that may put them at increased risk for HIV. Therefore, social workers must incorporate sexual risk within routine assessments when providing services to clients. To achieve this goal, training may be necessary to increase comfort among providers to address sexual risks among older clients. Social service agencies, in turn, must implement service and policy changes in order to mandate such assessments and provide staff with training opportunities.

Further, we anticipate that service providers will benefit from recognizing the cultural implications of this study within their practice. As stated previously, many layers of culture are addressed in this study, including cultural issues related to age, ethnicity and socioeconomic status. Although many of the women in this study recognize the effectiveness of condoms and believe that partners would approve of using condoms, these findings support the need for skill-building activities including condom negotiation. Such skills should be taught in settings that utilize appropriate resource materials, language and context in order to be effective among mature minority women. When working with African American communities and other communities of color, an understanding of specific behavioral contexts, such as the "down low," may be helpful in assessing social service needs. Further, social service providers must recognize the potential for increased risk behaviors among women living in impoverished and rural areas such as exchanging sex for something of value. It is imperative to implement practice, service and policy changes to accommodate the needs of these clients as well as the training needs of the social service providers that work with this underserved population.

There are limitations to the generalizability of this study's results. First, there is bias inherent in self-reported survey data, which may result an in over or under reporting of sensitive information such as sexual behavior (Catania, Gibson, Chitwood, & Coates, 1990). Second, potential limitations imposed by a cross-sectional research study design and a sample of convenience must be considered when generalizing results to other populations. Third, we surveyed women living in rural counties. This group of older women may be different from women living in larger, urban settings.

Despite the study limitations, this study along with previous research (Williams & Donnelly, 2002; Winningham et al., 2003; Wright, Drost, Caserta, & Lund, 1998) suggests that older adults are at increasing risk for HIV. Public health strategies to prevent HIV among this cohort are needed to prevent a rise in the epidemic among this age group. While we know a great deal about factors associated with risk and risk reduction among younger populations (Carey et al., 2000; Kelly & Kalichman, 2002; O'Leary, DiClemente, & Aral, 1997; Sterk, Theall, & Elifson, 2003), we know virtually nothing about how those models will work in this older age group. Prevention research is urgently needed to delineate age-appropriate messages and consider the contextual factors of older adults so that effective prevention interventions can be developed for older adults.

REFERENCES

Airhihenbuwa, C.O., DiClemente, R.J., Wingood, G.M., & Lowe, A. (1992). HIV/ AIDS education and prevention among African-Americans: A focus on culture. *AIDS Education and Prevention, 4*(3), 267-276.

Bachanas, P.J., Morris, M.K., Lewis-Gess, J.K., Sarett-Cuasay, E.J., Sirl, K., Ries, J.K., & Sawyer, M.K. (2002). Predictors of risky sexual behavior in African American adolescent girls: Implications for prevention interventions. *Journal of Pediatric Psychology, 27*(6), 519-530.

Binson, D., Pollack, L., & Catania, J. (1997). AIDS-related risk behaviors and safer sex practices of women in midlife and older in the United States: 1990 to 1992. *Health Care for Women International, 18,* 343-354.

Carey, M.P., Braaten, L.S., Maisto, S.A., Gleason, J.R., Forsyth, A.D., Durant, L.E., & Jaworski, B.C. (2000). Using information, motivational enhancement, and skills training to reduce the risk of HIV infection for low-income urban women: A second randomized clinical trial. *Health Psychology, 19*(1), 3-11.

Catania, J.A., Gibson, D.R., Chitwood, D.D., & Coates, T.J. (1990). Methodological problems in AIDS behavioral research: Influences on measurement error and participation bias in studies of sexual behavior. *Psychological Bulletin, 108*(3), 363-382.

Catania, J., Turner, H., Kegeles, S., Stall, R., Pollack, L., & Coates, T. (1989). Older Americans and AIDS: Transmission risks and primary prevention research needs. *The Gerontologist, 29*(3), 373-381.

Centers for Disease Control and Prevention. (2000). CDC *HIV/AIDS Surveillance Year-End 1999 Report,* 11 (2).

Centers for Disease Control and Prevention. (2001). CDC *HIV/AIDS Surveillance Year-End 2000 Report,* 12 (2).

Centers for Disease Control and Prevention. (2002). CDC *HIV/AIDS Surveillance Year-End 2001 Report,* 13 (2).

Center for Disease Control and Prevention (2003). Advancing HIV prevention: New strategies for a changing epidemic-United States, 2003. *Morbidity and Mortality Weekly Report, 52*(15), 329-33.

Cornelius, L.J., Okundaye, J.N., & Manning, M.C. (2000). Human Immunodeficiency Virus-related risk behavior among African American females. *Journal of the National Medical Association, 92*(4), 183-195.

Crosby, R.A., Yarber, W.L., DiClemente, R.J., Wingood, G.M., & Meyerson, B. (2002). HIV-associated histories, perceptions, and practices among low-income African American women: Does rural residence matter? *American Journal of Public Health, 92*(4), 655-659.

DeCarlo, P. (1997). *What are rural HIV prevention needs?* University of California San Francisco, Center for AIDS Prevention Studies and the AIDS Research Institute.

DiClemente, R.J. & Wingood, G.M. (1995). A randomized controlled trial of an HIV sexual risk reduction intervention for young African American women. *JAMA, 274*(16), 1271-1276.

Gielen, A.C, Faden, R.R., O'Campo, P., Kass, N., & Anderson, J. (1994). Women's protective sexual behaviors: A test of the Health Belief Model. *AIDS Education and Prevention, 6*(1), 1-11.

Hader, S.L., Smith, D.K., Moore, J.S., & Holmberg, S.D. (2001). HIV infection in women in the United States: Status at the millenium. *Journal of the American Medical Association*, 285(9), 1186-1192.

Hochbaum, G.M. (1958). *Public participation in medical screening programs: A sociopsychological study.* (Public Health Service, PHS Publication 572). Washington, DC: U.S. Government Printing Office.

Holmes, R., Fawal, H., Moon, T.D., Cheeks, J., Coleman, J., Woernle, C., & Vermund, S.H. (1997). Acquired Immunodeficiency Syndrome in Alabama: Special concerns for black women. *Southern Medical Journal, 90*(7), 1186-1192.

Kelly, J.A. & Kalichman, S.C. (2002). Behavioral research in HIV/AIDS primary and secondary prevention: Recent advances and future directions. *Journal of Consulting & Clinical Psychology*, 70(3), 626-639.

Kline, A., & VanLandingham, M. (1994). HIV-infected women and sexual risk reduction: The relevance of existing models of behavior change. *AIDS Education and Prevention*, 6(5), 390-402.

Lee, H., Ganges, L., Cross, H., & Garner, J. (1999). *Racial and ethnic disparities in HIV+ clients aged 50 and over.* Abstract submitted to the American Public Health Association Meeting, Boston, MA.

Moore, L.W., & Amburgey, L.B. (2000). Older adults and HIV. *AORN Journal, 71*(4), 873-876.

Nokes, K.M. (1996). *HIV/AIDS and the Older Adult.* New York: Taylor & Francis.

O'Leary, A., DiClemente, R.J., & Aral, S.O. (1997). Reflections on the design and reporting of STD/HIV behavioral intervention research. *AIDS Education & Prevention*, 9(1, suppl), 1-14.

Ory, M.G., & Mack, K.A. (1998). Middle-aged and older people with AIDS: Trends in national surveillance rates, transmission routes, and risk factors. *Research on Aging*, 20(6), 653-663.

Peterson, J., Wingood, G., DiClemente, R., DeCarlo, P., & Quirk, K. (1999). *What are African Americans' HIV prevention needs?* University of California San Francisco, Center for AIDS Prevention Studies and the AIDS Research Institute.

Riley, J.H. (1997). HIV/AIDS and the elderly. In F. Safford & G. Krell (Eds.). *Gerontology for Health Professionals: A Practice Guide* (pp. 162-178). Washington, DC: NASW Press.

Rosenstock, I.M. (1960). What research in motivation suggests for public health. *American Journal of Public Health*, 50, 295-301.

Rosenstock, I.M. (1966). Why people use health services. *Milbank Memorial Fund Quarterly*, 44, 94-124.

Rosenstock, I.M. (1974). Historical origins of the health belief model. *Health Education Monographs*, 2, 328-335.

Rural Center for the Study and Promotion of HIV/STD Prevention. (1996). *HIV/AIDS in rural America* (No. 8). Indiana University and Purdue University.

South Carolina Department of Health and Environmental Control. (2001). *HIV/AIDS Surveillance Report.*

St. Lawrence, J.S., Eldridge, G.D., Reitman, D., Little, C.E., Shelby, M.C., & Brasfield, T.L. (1998). Factors influencing condom use among African American women: Implications for risk reduction interventions. *American Journal of Community Psychology*, 26(1), 7-28.

Sterk, C.E., Theall, K.P., & Elifson, K.W. (2003). Effectiveness of a risk reduction intervention among African American women who use crack cocaine. *AIDS Education & Prevention*, 15(1), 15-32.

Sternberg, S. (March 15, 2001). The danger of living "down low": Black men who hide their bisexuality can put women at risk. *USA Today*, Arlington Virginia: D.01.

Stokes, M.E., Davis, C.S., & Koch, G.G. (1995). *Categorical Data Analysis Using the SAS System*. Cary, North Carolina: SAS Institute Inc.

Timmons, S.M. & Sowell, R.L. (1999). Perceived HIV-related sexual risks and prevention practices of African American women in the southeastern United States. *Health Care for Women International*, 20, 579-591.

United States Census Bureau. 2001. *Current Population Survey*.

Voelker, R. (1998). Rural communities struggle with AIDS. *Journal of the American Medical Association*, 279, 5-6.

Whipple, B. & Scura, K. (1996). The overlooked epidemic: HIV in older adults. *American Journal of Nursing*, 96 (2), 23-29.

Williams, E. & Donnelly, J. (2002). Older Americans and AIDS: Some guidelines for prevention. *Social Work*, 47(2), 105-110.

Wingood, G.M., & DiClemente, R.J. (1996). HIV sexual risk reduction interventions for women: A review. *American Journal of Preventive Medicine*, 12(3), 209-217.

Wingood, G.M., & DiClemente, R.J. (1998). Gender-related correlates and predictors of consistent condom use among young adult African-American women: A prospective analysis. *International Journal of STD & AIDS*, 9(3), 139-145.

Winiarski, K. (June 25, 2000). Columbia in top 5 of AIDS cases. *The State*.

Winningham, A.L., Corwin, S.J., Moore, C.G., Richter, D.L., Sargent, R., & Gore-Felton, C. (2003). *The Changing Age of HIV: Sexual Risk Among Older African American Women Living in Rural Communities*. In submission.

Wright, S.D., Drost, M., Caserta, M.S., & Lund, D.A. (1998). Older adults and HIV/AIDS: Implications for educators. *Gerontology & Geriatrics Education*, 18(4), 3-21.

Midlife Women with HIV:
Health, Social, and Economic Factors
Shaping Their Futures

Sharon M. Keigher, PhD, ACSW
Patricia E. Stevens, RN, PhD, FAAN
Sandra K. Plach, RN, PhD

SUMMARY. Women are the fastest growing population infected with HIV. They are more impoverished, less healthy, and they succumb to AIDS faster than men. Even in Wisconsin, a relatively low prevalence state, HIV/AIDS is a significant cause of morbidity and death for women, especially women of color. However, with improved antiretroviral medi-

---

Sharon M. Keigher, PhD, ACSW, is Professor at the Helen Bader School of Social Welfare, University of Wisconsin-Milwaukee.

Patricia E. Stevens, RN, PhD, FAAN, is Professor and Sandra K. Plach, PhD, is Assistant Professor at the College of Nursing, University of Wisconsin-Milwaukee.

Address correspondence to: Dr. Sharon M. Keigher, Helen Bader School of Social Welfare, University of Wisconsin-Milwaukee, P.O. Box 786, Milwaukee, WI 53212 (E-mail: keigher@uwm.edu).

This research is supported by grant number NIH RO1 NR04840, National Institutes of Health, National Institute for Nursing Research, Principal Investigator, Patricia E. Stevens.

An early version of this paper was presented at the 55th Annual Scientific Meetings of the Gerontological Society of America, Washington, DC, November 2002.

[Haworth co-indexing entry note]: "Midlife Women with HIV: Health, Social, and Economic Factors Shaping Their Futures." Keigher, Sharon M., Patricia E. Stevens, and Sandra K. Plach. Co-published simultaneously in *Journal of HIV/AIDS & Social Services* (The Haworth Press) Vol. 3, No. 1, 2004, pp. 43-58; and: *Midlife and Older Adults and HIV: Implications for Social Service Research, Practice, and Policy* (ed: Cynthia Cannon Poindexter, and Sharon M. Keigher) The Haworth Press, Inc., 2004, pp. 43-58. Single or multiple copies of this article are available for a fee from The Haworth Document Delivery Service [1-800-HAWORTH, 9:00 a.m. - 5:00 p.m. (EST). E-mail address: docdelivery@haworthpress.com].

cations and clinical care, many women diagnosed today with HIV will live into old age. What are their prospects for "successful aging?"

This essay presents qualitative data on 9 midlife Wisconsin women living with HIV to speculate about the probable trajectories and outcomes of their life-courses, highlighting their key security and longevity challenges. Financial resources, social support, health care and health needs will be critical to their prospects for survival. Only by strengthening basic social provisions for many marginalized groups in the United States will women with HIV have the prospect of sharing a future of "successful aging" that many other Americans take for granted. *[Article copies available for a fee from The Haworth Document Delivery Service: 1-800-HAWORTH. E-mail address: <docdelivery@haworthpress.com> Website: <http://www.HaworthPress.com> © 2004 by The Haworth Press, Inc. All rights reserved.]*

KEYWORDS. Older women, HIV/AIDS, midlife women, health care, social support, income security, qualitative research

An estimated 18.9 percent of Americans with AIDS, close to 90,000, were aged 50 and older at the end of 2000 (Centers for Disease Control and Prevention [CDC], 2003). The majority of these are men, but as incidence of HIV among women increases in successively younger and younger age cohorts, the proportion of women among older people with AIDS is increasing. HIV-infected women tend to be disadvantaged by poverty, unemployment, and lack of education, and subsequently have difficulty accessing adequate health care and social resources (Linn, Anema, Estrada, Cain, & Sharpe, 1996; Moneyham, Sowell, Seals, & Demi, 2000). Gender disparity is especially apparent relative to ethnicity and race. African-American women and Latinas represented 80 percent of AIDS cases reported in women in 2000 (CDC, 2002).

At this time in history, women with HIV/AIDS who are surviving to middle age share the experience of living with a stigmatizing disease and requiring medical treatment throughout the remainder of their lives (Levy, Ory, & Crystal, 2003). For almost two decades, the number of American women infected with HIV has continued to rise, and from 1985 to 1999 the number of AIDS cases among U.S. women more than tripled. Women now comprise 17 percent of persons with AIDS in the United States, and 25 percent of persons with HIV (CDC, 2002). The profile of HIV infection has changed in the same time period from an acute condition with a fatal outcome to a chronic disease characterized by health decline over many years (Lyon & Younger, 2001; Williams, 1997; Ungvarski, 1997). As a result of the newer combination anti-retroviral drug therapies in recent years, survival rates for women with HIV have improved so much that many can now expect to live into old age. Yet, their old age will likely include compromised health and functional abilities, and the social and financial effects of years of marginalization. What chances do they really have for sharing in the positive gains made by most older adults in recent years in our aging society? What are their prospects for "successful aging" (Rowe & Kahn, 1998, p. 38)?

In their upbeat assessment of the changing norms and expectations of midlife Americans, Rowe and Kahn define "successful aging" as the ability to maintain three key behaviors or characteristics of oneself from midlife forward (1998, p. 38). The first is avoidance of diseases and disease-related disability. The second is maintenance of high mental and physical functioning. And finally, one must remain actively engaged in life through both valued and contributory activities and satisfying social relationships with people and living environments. These dimensions interact within a kind of hierarchical order, in that disease may certainly trump functional abilities, and erosion of functional powers usually circumscribe one's ability to work and socialize. But these are not entirely predictive in that order. Examples abound of older adults adapting successfully to chronic illnesses through good medical care and conscientious personal efforts, caring for themselves, adapting their daily routines, and maintaining social relationships and commitments to other engagements with life (Corbin & Straus, 1991). Social connectedness has distinct effects for survival (House, 1988), and the experience of being supported has direct positive effects on health itself (Kahn & Antonucci, 1980). The feeling that one is "cared for, loved, esteemed and a member of a network of mutual obligations" can protect adults from the effects of stressful life events and even lead to experiencing less pain, faster recovery, and better adherence to medical regimens (Rowe & Kahn, 1998, p. 157).

Since the indexing of Social Security in the early 1970s, elders' living standards have greatly increased, contributing to these improved probabilities for security. Rowe and Kahn (1998) caution, however, that by the early 1990s only 15 percent of adults over 65 had any financial assets beyond their home equity and Social Security (p. 186). Furthermore, 12 percent were still living below the poverty level, suggesting the fundamental importance of universal social protection and continuing opportunities for income production for a large share of older adults.

In this illustrated essay we address the prospects for successful aging of women living with HIV/AIDS who are now in midlife. We speculate about what aging may do to them, given their current health status and socioeconomic circumstances. While these speculations are sensitized by research data, they are not meant to be a report of findings. Rather, we use narrative excerpts from the stories of nine midlife women who participated in our research to illustrate the real-life contexts in which HIV-infected women find themselves. We draw our cases from Wisconsin, a state with relatively strong publicly supported social services and income benefit levels. Our aim is to illustrate for practitioners and policymakers the complex set of needs women with HIV will bring to health care and social service systems as they age. Our argument about the future of midlife women with HIV is meant as a challenge to social work practice, the aging network, and the future of U.S. social policy.

Variability in education, employment, income, substance use, care-taking of children, sexuality, severity of symptoms, and social support all affect the chances for successful aging of midlife women. Each aspect of a woman's life creates for her an identity that may or may not facilitate attachment to other people, services, and other resources; the diversity of her attachments can have life-sustaining, or life-threatening, implications.

What are the critical vulnerabilities confronting midlife women with HIV? Our analysis utilizes Rowe and Kahn's theory of "successful aging" which emphasizes the criticality of health, social support, and economic well-being (p. 38). Their framework allows us to identify specific health, social, and economic barriers to securing infected women's lives as they grow into old age and thus suggest ways of mobilizing to ensure successful aging for women living with HIV/AIDS. Unless addressed now by practitioners and policy makers, these barriers will surely limit women's survival chances as well as their capacities to live well. If ours is a caring society, these challenges are certainly surmountable.

The nine life stories we use to illustrate our argument are taken from a longitudinal qualitative study we have been conducting since 2000 with 55 Wisconsin women who have HIV. We have interviewed each woman ten times over two years to explore the impact HIV has had in her life. Women have described their health needs in rich detail, how they deal with symptoms, when and under what conditions treatment regimens become difficult, how they conduct their private lives, and where they access health care and social services. To assure strictest confidentiality of this information, our university Institutional Review Board reviewed and approved the study. In the course of approximately 20 hours of interview time with each woman, we have learned a great deal about the context in which she lives. The women portrayed here are those in our sample who were age 50 or older when the interviews began. Each is identified by a pseudonym in the following stories. Table 1 outlines the basic socio-demographics of these nine women.

THE STORIES

We open our discussion of the stories of these nine midlife women by examining in turn their experiences with illness, health care, social roles, social support, and financial security. From these experiences we speculate in our discussion about practice and policy toward meeting their needs as they grow older with HIV/AIDS into the future.

TABLE 1. Sociodemographic and Health Characteristics of Women with HIV (Ranked by Monthly Income)

Participant (Case #)	Race/ Ethnicity	Age	HIV Source	HIV Status	Diagnosis (Year)	Relationship Status	Children/ Relationship	Housing	Monthly Income
Paula	White	51	Sexual	HIV	1986	Divorced	0	Own	$2,650
Mitsy (3)	White	50	IV Drug	AIDS	1989	Single	0	Rent	$1,020
Fran (4)	White	53	Sexual	HIV	1992	Widowed	1/Deceased	Rent	$1,000
Martina (1)	Latina	50	Sexual	AIDS	1992	Widowed	4/Close	Rent	$850
Sonny	Black	50	Sexual	AIDS	1995	Married	5/Close	Rent	$800
Mae (5)	Black	55	Sexual	HIV	1994	Divorced	3/Distant	Unstable	$666
Mildred	White	56	Sexual	HIV	1995	Married	2/Close	Rent	$628
Vanessa (2)	Black	54	IV Drug	AIDS	1989	Divorced	3/Distant	Nursing home	$30*
Gail	Black	50	Sexual	HIV	1996	Single	4/Distant	Unstable	$0

*Nursing home residents are allowed $30 per month from SSI for personal expenses. The balance of Vanessa's SSI is used for cost of the home and her care.

47

Illness

The 9 women ranged from 36 to 50 years old when they first tested positive for HIV; on average they've been infected for 7 years (ranging from 4 to 13 years). In the intervening years four of them progressed to AIDS, but all nine have contended with co-morbid health conditions as well, including hypertension, diabetes, depression and hepatitis. All nine had been on anti-retroviral medications at one time or another, although most had struggled to adapt to these regimens, suffered side effects, and had taken drug holidays. Three had quit taking HIV medications altogether at the time of our first interviews. Substance misuse had been a problem for five of the nine; and two, Gail and Mae, continued to smoke crack and engage in problematic drinking.

Martina deals with many complicating co-morbidities. She contends with more co-morbidities than the other women, but unlike some of them, she has also received continuous health care that appears to have extended her life (see Case 1).

Health Care

Three of the nine women have received little or no health care since being diagnosed with HIV, a pattern consistent with the lack of care they had had previously. One of these three, Vanessa, died during the study, but she received end-of-life care in a nursing home during her last several months (see Case 2).

CASE 1. Martina: A Multitude of Maladies

Martina has been diagnosed with bi-polar illness, diabetes, hypertension, congestive heart failure, asthma, Hepatitis B, arthritis, and sleep apnea. She also has back and ankle pain from old fractures and gynecological problems. She has been near death several times with AIDS-related pneumonias. She has had numerous side-effects from HIV medications, and lots of difficulty adhering to treatment regimens.

A 50 year old Latina from Puerto Rico, Martina grew up in New York before coming to Wisconsin 20 years ago with her small children to escape an abusive husband. When diagnosed with HIV in 1992, she was told she had only two years to live. Her second husband deserted her and she "went crazy," "did a lot of drugs," became deeply depressed and suicidal, and blamed God for her situation. She subsequently became involved with another man she loved very much, but they stopped having intercourse when they learned he was infected. She cared for him until he died from AIDS in 1999, and is still deeply saddened at losing him. In addition, her strong involvement as a consumer representative and advocate at an AIDS service organization has brought her close to many more persons with AIDS, many of whom have died. Her own health problems have forced her to reduce this involvement in recent years and now she focuses mainly on getting her last son through high school.

HIV is "voodoo" in the Hispanic community and Martina feels that she and her partner had a spell put on them. While her spiritual beliefs keep her going, Martina continues to feel anger toward God for bringing AIDS into her life.

CASE 2. Vanessa: Homelessness and Health Care

Raised in Mississippi, Vanessa married a man who abused her. She eventually raised her three children alone, doing kitchen work when she could get it, and otherwise supporting her family on AFDC. For her last 20 years she was addicted to drugs and alcohol. She sometimes lived with a daughter, but eventually became estranged from all her children. She spent many years living in shelters or on the streets in several large Midwestern cities. She never had health insurance, receiving health care intermittently at emergency rooms, and community supported clinics and hospitals.

Gail's and Mae's health care use, both before and after their diagnoses, mirror Vanessa's, as did their lifelong poverty, inadequate housing, and involvements with abusive men. Diagnosed in 1996, Gail has relied solely on hospital emergency rooms and clinics for homeless people. Her only health coverage has been the county General Assistance Medical Program (GAMP), which covers care at these free clinics. Diagnosed in 1994, Mae has never received regular care for her HIV either, despite being intermittently employed. When she entered the study, she was about to pass her probationary employment period as a nurse's aide, which would have made her eligible for health care benefits. However, before this milestone occurred, she was fired for what she believes was discrimination because of her HIV status.

Five of the women have histories of injection drug use, although only two (Mitsy and Vanessa) point to injection drug use as their route of infection. Mitsy had quit using on her own before she contracted HIV, but Vanessa continued using until admitted to a nursing home at the end of her life. Vanessa, Mae and Gail (the three African-American respondents with the least education and incomes) all continued using drugs while on the streets. Martina had also used injection drugs, but was able to quit with the help of drug treatment. These various trajectories suggest that education, income, supportive children, and other social resources may help women reach recovery, both before and after HIV infection, but also that being African-American in the U.S. may exacerbate vulnerability to addiction as well as HIV.

In generally better circumstances than Vanessa, Gail, and Mae, four of the nine, Mildred, Fran, Sonny, and Martina, indicated that they have adequate access to health care. Living on Social Security Disability in a small community, Mildred had difficulty finding specialty HIV care and, because of several co-morbidities, even with Medicare and the Ryan White AIDS Drug Assistance Program (ADAP), has struggled to afford her many medications. Fran, on the other hand, has health insurance through steady employment, but chooses not to utilize health care more than getting an annual physical. She is relatively free of HIV-related symptoms and attributes this to her reliance on naturopathic remedies, healthy nutrition and exercise. Both Sonny and Martina are covered by Medicare and Medicaid, receive health care through medical managed care networks, and have complex health needs. Sonny received care at a

VA medical center for several years, but was dissatisfied with its quality and subsequently switched providers. Now, even with her own infectious disease, physician and close case management, she has been unable to adapt to the side effects of her HIV medications, difficulties compounded by her gynecological problems and depression. Martina receives close case management at a multi-disciplinary university hospital HIV clinic, but like Sonny, also struggles with medication side effects along with her many co-morbidities.

The remaining two, Paula and Mitsy, receive private medical care, which they consider excellent. Both use Medicare, Paula's supplemented by private insurance from her former employer, and Mitsy's supplemented by Medicaid. Mitsy's present medical care, however, highlights one of the significant failures of American health policy. Unable to qualify for Social Security Disability and Medicare in 1993 when she became very ill with AIDS, she "finally" became eligible only after her kidneys failed (see Case 3).

Social Roles and Social Support

In midlife, as part of normal aging, women generally begin shedding the familial roles and responsibilities they assumed in early adulthood. But research confirms the continuing importance of social roles for women with HIV, who often feel guilty about what their families go through because of their diagnosis (Goggin et al., 2001; van Servellen et al., 1998). Some confide that one of the worst aspects of the discovery of their HIV infection was their subsequent loss of vital roles and relationships–their ability to work, bear and raise children, and enjoy present and future sexual relationships.

Women who are married or live with a partner report higher levels of anxiety and more HIV-related symptoms than women who are single (Goggin et

CASE 3. Mitsy: "Kidney failure was the best thing that happened to me."

"In 1989 I started getting a lot of yeast infections and mouth thrush," says Mitsy. "It was my dentist that said. 'I hate to tell you this, but I think you better get checked out for HIV.' He was very hip to the signs of it." Mitsy was already trying to give up the injection drugs that had come to rule her life for eight years. After her HIV diagnosis she managed to get clean, make new friends, and finish her teaching degree. In 1992, however, she became very ill with AIDS. She was ruled ineligible for Social Security Disability, although, "I couldn't even get off my couch."

It was not until complications from the treatment of her Hepatitis C caused kidney failure that she qualified for Social Security Disability. In retrospect she says, "When my kidneys failed, that was the best thing that happened to me. I was finally able to get Medicare." She was referred to a kidney specialist who still coordinates her care, working closely with an HIV specialist who was assigned to her. Mitsy feels that the dialysis she receives three days per week provides excellent contact with a whole team of health care providers. Reflecting on her care, "I'm surrounded by people living with HIV who are constantly complaining about their health coverage, and it makes me feel bad because I have absolutely no problems. I have the best doctors. I can go anywhere I want for anything with Medicare and Medicaid."

al., 2001). It may be that the demands of carrying multiple roles of spouse/ partner, homemaker, and/or mother, and in some cases care-giving for another HIV-infected person, is particularly difficult when sick and struggling to manage one's own health. In a cross-sectional study of HIV-infected women, women working full-time had less anxiety and fewer HIV-symptoms than women who were unemployed, suggesting that employed women may have greater financial security and other resources to offset the stress effects of HIV infection (Sowell et al., 1997). Three of the women enjoy part-time employment in service professions, work that is very meaningful to each. The other six women are either physically unable to work or have never had marketable skills.

Having a partner is one route to security for women, although only two of the nine, Mildred and Sonny, are currently in partnered relationships. Martina, Fran, and Sonny had each previously cared for a partner who died of AIDS, leaving each of them emotionally exhausted. Another potential source of support in adulthood is one's own parents. If parents are still living and available as women reach midlife, however, these relationships typically involve reciprocal duties. Sonny, Mitsy, and Gail each still have a living parent who knows and accepts their HIV illness, and provides emotional support. But others fear that disclosure of this stigmatized illness to parents may upset their balance of mutual social support. Mildred, who was diagnosed after her mother died, felt relieved that "She never found out I had HIV, thank God." Fran, who lives in her parents' neighborhood, has never disclosed her HIV status to them, although they are very supportive of her, and even volunteer with her helping AIDS patients, Fran is leaving her own status ambiguous as long as she is asymptomatic to avoid dealing with her parents' reaction. Paula's parents are deceased, and Mae has been estranged from her family of origin since her adolescence. Even when completely supportive, parents, as well as partners, will be able to provide only decreasing levels of social support as these women get older.

The key source of social support for most midlife adults gradually becomes their grown children. We expected those with close relationships with their children to have better social support and life chances generally than those who do not. However, recent research on the life-time costs of raising children raises doubts about any financial "advantages" of having children (Crittenden, 2003). Martina, Sonny, and Mildred speak affectionately of their children. Martina's grown sons have been incarcerated and have had difficulty settling down, but she supports them emotionally and is very close to her teenaged son still living at home. Sonny's children and grandchildren live in distant cities and she goes to great lengths to visit and communicate regularly with them. Mildred's children, who live nearby, help her out occasionally. These ties of affection, including links with future grandchildren, increase the probabilities of receiving social support and even intimate personal care in the future. However, unless one has daughters living nearby (who typically provide intimate care), daily personal care is still unlikely to be available.

For the rest of our sample, ties with children either never existed or have been broken. Three of the nine–Mitsy, Paula, and Fran–have no living children. Vanessa, Mae, and Gail have grown children with whom they have had conflicts or become estranged. Mae, for example, considers herself a loner and isolates herself from nearly everyone except occasional sexual partners. Gail's four children strongly disapprove of her drinking and drugging, but she stays with them intermittently, occasionally providing child care in return.

Some of the women with more education and financial resources, who have neither partners nor children, have created supportive social structures for themselves. Mitsy has several siblings and other relatives who visit often. She, Paula, and Fran rely on sets of supportive friends with whom they enjoy talking, sharing activities, and, on rare occasions, traveling. These involve deep commitments and in return, the women can count on these friends when they are sick. Fran has developed a whole network of new friends through her volunteer work for an AIDS service organization, although these relationships are somewhat bittersweet (see Case 4).

Financial Security

All of the women have experienced combinations of personal and economic losses. For several, poor financial circumstances before they contracted HIV precluded their mobilizing any but the most basic resources for themselves after their diagnoses. Those whose exposure to HIV was related to risks they had taken just to survive now have the slimmest chances of all of ever living well. For instance, Mae, Gail, and Vanessa, for periods of their lives, had exchanged sex for drugs, money, a place to stay, or as a means of providing for their children.

Mae expresses determination to continue "making it" on her own (see Case 5). She and Fran are the only women among our nine who are still working and receiving no government income. (Gail was not receiving government assistance either, but she no longer had a job). Mae and Gail (and Vanessa until she died) stayed transiently with relatives or acquaintances, in shelters, or, sometimes, on the streets. Intermittently they stayed with men who sometimes pro-

CASE 4. Fran: Being of Service to Friends

"My spouse died in 1997 from complications due to AIDS. A lot of my friends in the women's group have died, too. I was lucky I was able to be with them in the end. I volunteer at hospice. And a lot of friends of mine have gone through there and passed away there. It's actually kind of . . . I don't want to say comforting, but it makes it easier to face what I have to go through, being able to be of service to them in their last moments. I think if I didn't have something like that, that would be harder. I think I'd be more dwelling on my disease and things like that, but because I have so much to do with helping other people and keeping busy I don't dwell on the negative part of having HIV. I dwell more on the positive part."

CASE 5. Mae: "An old woman out there . . . trying to hustle"

Diagnosed with HIV in 1995, Mae, now age 55, has never taken HIV medications because she feels "they only result in a longer life of poor health." Tough, independent, and lonely, she participated in the study because "I need someone to talk to." Employed off and on as a nursing assistant, she was living in the basement of an acquaintance's home, hoping to move to her own apartment when she has saved up enough for deposits, moving expenses, and furniture. She has few friends, no contact with her children, and smokes crack cocaine occasionally to keep up her energy.

Mae grew up fast in Mississippi as the oldest of nine children. When their mother went to work, Mae got the others off to school. Her mother occasionally beat her with a hairbrush, and by age 12, Mae was doing all the cooking, cleaning and caring for the younger siblings. Mae left school in tenth grade to clean in a "nice white lady's home." She saved her money and, at age 18, ran away. Mae did housekeeping and personal care, married a Navy man, and had her first child at age 28, with two more in quick succession. She raised them on AFDC, but provided them a good home and they even "had a car." Married four times and divorced three, her husbands beat her, but Mae says that "is the black woman's life."

In her 40s, when her kids were teenagers, Mae began smoking crack cocaine. Within a short time, she lost all her possessions, became homeless, and started exchanging sex for drugs. During that time she lived "on the streets," sleeping in shelters when she could, and using food pantries. Then, at about age 50, "I just stopped using." It was just too hard, she says, "being an old woman out there . . . trying to hustle."

vided for them. These three had the poorest financial circumstances at the time of the interviews, and only Mae had earned income that year. None of them had health insurance, although Vanessa received SSI and Medicaid after being admitted to the nursing home where she subsequently died.

For Martina, Mildred, and Sonny, Supplemental Security Income (SSI), the means tested federal benefit, provides their only incomes–from $628 to $950 per month. Each receives some rental assistance (Housing for Persons with AIDS or HUD Section 8) for their modest apartments. (Unfortunately, both Mildred and Sonny believe the housing agencies disclosed their diagnoses to their neighbors, creating hostility toward them.) These three depend on food pantries, or on partners and other household members to get by.

Paula's, Mitsy's, and Fran's economic circumstances are better, and they have more stable housing. Only two, Paula and Mitsy, receive Social Security Disability (SSD), the earned entitlement benefit. Paula also has an inheritance from her parents as well as a company pension for a monthly income of about $2,650. She lives comfortably in her own condominium in an upscale urban neighborhood. Mitsy receives about $700 in SSD per month. She supplements this by substitute teaching, although the SSD earnings limits preclude her from earning more than about $320 per month, and losing her SSD benefit would jeopardize her Medicare and Medicaid eligibility. Mitsy rents a small duplex apartment in a safe, pleasant neighborhood, with the help of some Section 8 rental assistance. Fran works four days a week at a service job through which she receives health insurance, and lives in a relative's flat for which she pays very low rent. With these basics covered, Fran gets by without any government benefits.

Transportation also tells an economic story. Only Sonny, Paula, and Fran have cars they drive, and Mildred's husband drives her when necessary, or she would be homebound. Mitsy pays a carpool or takes buses to work, and rides a medical van to dialysis. Gail gets rides from relatives sometimes; she and Mae are quite resourceful, also using the city buses, and walking. Martina rarely leaves her home.

Several of the women's incomes had already been reduced dramatically when they had to give up employment because of their health. Nearly all had experienced income loss and subsequent dislocations when a partner or other co-residing relative died, children grew up and left home, or rents increased beyond their means. For these women, the security, privacy, and comfort of a stable home is already the high priority it would be to much older adults (Benjamin, 1996). The Department of Housing and Urban Development estimated in the early 1990s that one-third to one-half of Persons with AIDS in the U.S. is homeless or in imminent danger of losing their homes (DHUD, n.d.). Stable housing promotes continuity in the use of comprehensive healthcare and improved health status, as it did for Sonny. It promotes sobriety and decreased use of illicit drugs, as it did for Martina, and for some, like Mitsy, even a return to productive work and social activities. It is a prerequisite for receiving and adhering to complex medication regimens. In the future as they age, unless Social Security benefits increase substantially, all but one of these women will need rental assistance or very affordable housing. Dramatic increases in our nation's presently tiny stock of service-enhanced housing will be needed for women like Mae, Gail, and Vanessa whose histories of mental illness, substance misuse, and homelessness frequently dissipate with lots of support and close case-management.

THE FUTURE

Some of these women will certainly live to celebrate their 65th birthdays, the milestone at which working Americans can retire on Social Security. But none of them will be "retiring." Of the three who were working during our interviews (Fran, Mae, and Mitsy), Mae was subsequently fired, and Mitsy was working to supplement her Social Security Disability check. Fran will continue working as long as she can, but since she has already reduced her work to part-time, she worries that her income will not keep pace with the cost-of-living. If she works until age 65, her Social Security benefits will be no greater than if she quits and qualifies for SSD earlier. And Mae, unlikely to ever earn 40 quarters of FICA contributions, is unlikely to qualify for Social Security, not at age 62 nor when she becomes disabled. Instead, Mae will qualify only for SSI, the smaller means-tested benefit for disabled persons with less than

$2,000 in assets. SSI has, or will, qualify all the women (except Paula) for Medicaid, and Medicaid will be their lifeline to all their vital medications, hospitalizations, medical care, in-home personal care, and if necessary, nursing home care.

If these women's stories can suggest the reality for others, we can speculate that women who grow older with HIV in the future will be highly challenged financially, proving once again the arguments that have been made about the feminization of poverty among the elderly (Stone, 1989; Barusch, 1994). Even the slightest tinkering with deductibles or premiums, or reductions in Medicaid benefits or the Ryan White program will require these women to choose between receiving care and being able to afford a balanced diet, remain in their homes, and continue valuable connection to their own loved ones. Those without health care coverage now, like Mae and Gail, will require aggressive outreach, case management, and substance abuse treatment to stabilize their lives and prevent possible infection of others. Social workers will be expected to know how to help them stop using illicit drugs, find jobs, and get their sex partners to use condoms.

But where will these women live? Structural racism has already isolated the five minority women in our sample to the poorest, highly segregated central city neighborhoods where they and their families have the least job opportunities and greatest everyday health risks. The city continues to hemorrhage manufacturing jobs and its poverty rate rose by 14.3 percent between 2001 to 2002 and in the poorest neighborhoods, street violence deters women from getting vital exercise, and local convenience stores do not even carry fresh fruits and vegetables.

It is unlikely that any of these women will be safe living alone anyway, simply because of their fragile health. Yet few will be cared for by their children, either because they have none, or their children have died, moved away, are working all the time, or are simply unreliable. Even though many have supported and cared for sick and dying spouses, it is unlikely any will have partners, and fewer still will have daughters nearby to provide personal care.

Four of the women are already receiving housing assistance, and most will eventually need it. They may also need congregate housing (202 Supportive Housing for the Elderly), or even service-enhanced housing (Housing for People with AIDS, and Shelter Plus Care), if they are to maintain contact with friends and relatives. Social workers' input will be needed to advocate for, locate and design such housing to encourage positive social interaction among residents, between them and neighborhoods, facilitate support groups, and collaborate effectively with community organizations who must be welcomed. Without such housing those who have alienated their children will, like Vanessa, be exiled to nursing homes prematurely, simply because they need a place to stay.

In another decade most of these women will have lived on a "fixed income" for over 20 years. They will have accumulated few if any assets; only one will have ever owned a home. Few will have ever had a car, or even a savings account. None will have provided college for their children and few will have ever had a vacation away from home.

The security challenges facing them, and all low-income Baby Boomers, will have been greatly exacerbated by our federal government's unwillingness to address the eroding value of the minimum SSI and Social Security benefits. In the years since most of these women became HIV positive, Congress defeated a plan for universal health insurance that would have made them all eligible for comprehensive medical care. Despite the creation of new rental assistance programs, our overall supply of both affordable rental units and rental assistance declined dramatically throughout the 1980s and 1990s, simply because rising prosperity for higher income families drove up rents faster than the poorest families could afford (DHUD, 2002). Now in the early 21st century, state governments' fiscal crises preclude even maintaining basic universal services like public education and child welfare. In 2003, virtually all the states are fiscally unable to maintain even basic services. The "war on terrorism" and the suddenly voracious federal deficit could preclude for another generation the expansion of essential basic benefits for Americans with HIV/AIDS. Social workers need to hold federal and local elected officials accountable for this, using our moral authority to connect this erosion to the greater toll HIV will take if they deny it.

For the women we have described here, the financial cost of health care pales in comparison to the emotional cost to society of their deaths, which will be widely and deeply felt by persons who still depend on their sage advice, deep emotional resources, and courage, all honed through perseverance during the worst years of this epidemic. Some of them surely will die before getting "old," never receiving comprehensive health benefits, regular care, or effective treatment, despite living in a state only minimally impacted by HIV, which provides some of the best social care and benefits, in the richest country on earth.

Successful aging is a promising ideal for a "graying" nation, but until adequate income support and basic health care becomes a human right for all Americans, the financial and social survival challenges facing women with HIV will continue to supercede the ravages of the disease. With women's life chances so circumscribed by this infection, the economic and social features of being ill are at least as virulent as the virus itself.

The lives and circumstances of these women fall precisely within the responsibilities of social workers, case managers, and planners in AIDS service organizations and other institutions. The complications of their lives and the dilemmas they present are exacerbated by regressive and repressive social policies that have greatly disadvantaged women of color, women with children, and women who are poor. Changing societal demographics may create even more disadvantage for women in the future. Despite its becoming more challenging all the time, practitioners need to advocate locally and nationally for maintenance of the Ryan White Care Act and other supportive compensatory provisions: housing assistance, health care, outreach, substance abuse treatment, and strengthened basic income benefits.

REFERENCES

Barusch, A. S. (1994). *Older women in poverty: Private lives and public policies.* New York: Springer.

Benjamin, A. E. (1996). Trends among younger persons with disability or chronic disease. In R. H. Binstock, L. E. Cluff, & O. Von Mering (Eds.), *The future of long-term care: Social and policy issues* (pp. 75-95). Baltimore: Johns Hopkins Press.

CDC. (Centers for Disease Control & Prevention). (2002, March 23). *HIV/AIDS among US women: Minority and young women at continuing risk.* Retrieved April 25, 2002, from HIV Prevention Web Site: http://www.cdc.gov/hiv/pubs/facts/women.htm

CDC (Centers for Disease Control & Prevention). (2003). AIDS cases in adolescents and adults by age–United States, 1994-2000, *HIV/AIDS Surveillance Supplemental Report*, (9), 1-24.

Corbin, J. M., & Straus, A. L. (1991). A nursing model for chronic illness management based on the trajectory framework. *Scholarly Inquiry for Nursing Practice*, 5(3), 155-173.

Crittenden, A. (2003, Sept). Mothers most vulnerable. *The American Prospect, 14(8)*, 32.

DHUD (Department of Housing and Urban Development, n.d.). *HIV/AIDS Housing.* Retrieved online at: http://www.hud.gov:80/offices/cpd/aidshousing/index.cfm

DHUD (Department of Housing and Urban Development). (2002, July 11). Rental housing assistance–The worsening crisis: A Report to Congress on Worst Case Housing Needs, online at: http://www.huduser.org/publications/affhsg/worstcase00/ch3.html

Goggin, K., Catley, D., Brisco, S. T., Engelson, E. S., Rabkin, J. G., & Kotler, D. P. (2001, May). A female perspective on living with HIV disease, *Health & Social Work*, 26(2), 80-89.

House, J. S. (1988, July 29). Social relationships and health, *Science 241*: 540.

Kahn, R. L., & Antonucci, T. C. (1980). Convoys over the life course. In P. B. Baltes & O. G. Brimm (Eds.), *Life span development and behavior.* New York: Academic Press.

Levy, J. A. Ory, M. G., & Crystal, S. (2003, June). HIV/AIDS interventions for midlife and older adults: Current status and challenges. *Journal of Acquired Immune Deficiency Syndrome, 33* (Suppl. 2), S59-S67.

Linn, J. G., Anema, M. G., Estrada, J. J., Cain, V. A., & Sharpe, C. P. (1996). Self-appraised health, HIV infection, and depression in female clients of AIDS counseling centers. *AIDS Patient Care & Standards, 10*(4), 250-257.

Lyon, D. E., & Younger, J. B. (2001). Purpose in life and depressive symptoms in persons living with HIV disease. *Journal of Nursing Scholarship, 33*, 129-133.

Mack, K. & Ory, M.G. (2003). AIDS and older Americans at the end of the 20th century. *Journal of Acquired Immune Deficiency Syndrome, 33* (Suppl. 2), S68-S75.

Moneyham, L., Sowell, R., Seals, B., & Demi, A. (2000). Depressive symptoms among African American women with HIV disease. *Scholarly Inquiry for Nursing Practice: An International Journal, 14*, 9-39.

Rowe, J. W., & Kahn, K. A. (1998). *Successful aging.* Pantheon: New York.

Sowell, R. L., Seals, B. F., Moneyham, L., Demi, A., Cohen, L., & Brake, S. (1997). Quality of life in HIV-infected women in the Southeastern United States, *AIDS CARE, 9*, 501-512.

Stone, R. (1989). The feminization of poverty among the elderly. *Women's Studies Quarterly, 17*, 20-34.

Ungvarski, P. (1997). Adherence to prescribed HIV-1 protease inhibitors in the home setting. *Journal of the Association of Nurses in AIDS Care, 8, Supplement*, 37-45.

van Servellen, G., Sarna, L., Nyamathi, A., Padilla, G., Brecht, M., & Jablonski, K. J. (1998). Emotional distress in women with symptomatic HIV disease. *Issues in Mental Health Nursing, 19*, 173-189.

Williams, A. B. (1997). New horizons: Antiretroviral therapy in 1997. *Journal of the Association of Nurses in AIDS Care, 8*(4), 26-38.

Reconciling Successful Aging with HIV: A Biopsychosocial Overview

David E. Vance, PhD, MGS
F. Patrick Robinson, PhD, RN, ACRN

SUMMARY. As HIV is increasingly viewed as a chronic condition, primary care clinicians, case managers, and researchers must address the emerging implications of aging with this disease. Many aspects of HIV overlap with similar aspects of the aging process; however, a synthesis of topics related to both phenomena reveals some unique influences on disease prognosis, which affect the social, psychological, and medical well-being of persons aging with this disease. Fortunately, the gerontological literature is replete with theories, models, and examples of how to age successfully. This literature can inform the topic of aging with HIV in order to provide direction for research, interventions, and services. Trends found within both aging and HIV contexts are used to predict po-

David E. Vance, PhD, MGS, is currently a National Institute on Aging Postdoctoral Fellow at the Edward R. Roybal Center for Research in Applied Gerontology at the University of Alabama at Birmingham. Dr. Vance's research focuses on the treatment of cognitive decline in older adults.

F. Patrick Robinson, PhD, RN, ACRN, is currently a Biobehavioral Research Fellow in the College of Nursing at the University of Illinois at Chicago. Dr. Robinson's research program centers on treatment modalities to reduce cardiovascular risk in HIV-positive individuals with lipodystrophy.

Address correspondence to: David Vance, PhD, HMB 100, UAB, Birmingham, AL 35294-2100 (E-mail: devance@uab.edu).

[Haworth co-indexing entry note]: "Reconciling Successful Aging with HIV: A Biopsychosocial Overview." Vance, David E., and F. Patrick Robinson. Co-published simultaneously in *Journal of HIV/AIDS & Social Services* (The Haworth Press) Vol. 3, No. 1, 2004, pp. 59-78; and: *Midlife and Older Adults and HIV: Implications for Social Service Research, Practice, and Policy* (ed: Cynthia Cannon Poindexter, and Sharon M. Keigher) The Haworth Press, Inc., 2004, pp. 59-78. Single or multiple copies of this article are available for a fee from The Haworth Document Delivery Service [1-800-HAWORTH, 9:00 a.m. - 5:00 p.m. (EST). E-mail address: docdelivery@haworthpress.com].

tential difficulties in cognitive decline, depression, social withdrawal, financial planning, immune dysfunction, and mitochondria damage. To understand the biopsychosocial mechanisms surrounding successful aging with HIV, mitochondria damage is used to illustrate the dynamic effects of physical, psychological, and social functioning on each other. Interventions and questions for further research in successful aging with HIV are presented. *[Article copies available for a fee from The Haworth Document Delivery Service: 1-800-HAWORTH. E-mail address: <docdelivery@haworth press.com> Website: <http://www.HaworthPress.com> © 2004 by The Haworth Press, Inc. All rights reserved.]*

KEYWORDS. HIV/AIDS, successful aging, psychomotor, social support, mitochondria

The advent of Highly Active Antiretroviral Therapy (HAART) has dramatically decreased HIV-related mortality (Palella et al., 1998), giving rise to the possibility that those infected with HIV may reach older adulthood. This optimism is highlighted by the recent introduction of yet another new class of drugs called fusion inhibitors (Tashima & Carpenter, 2003). However, new infections are also contributing to the growing number of older adults with HIV.

Disease transmission has occurred in this group by different mechanisms. Based on 1997 CDC surveillance data on adults over 50, transmission via sexual contact represents the most prevalent type with gay/bisexual behavior representing 48% and heterosexual behavior representing 12%, followed by intravenous (IV) drug use comprising 17%, and blood transfusions accounting for 6% (Linsk, 2000). The dearth of information on aging with HIV may result partly from the misguided belief that older adults are not at risk for sexual contact or drug use; however, this is inaccurate. Slusher, Halman, Eshleman, and Ostrow (1993) found that 44% of homosexual men 60 and over reported multiple partners, rates that were similar in a 30 to 39 age group. Some older men who have sex with men may not identify themselves as homosexual, which only obfuscates the issues. Living in an age of Viagra has further increased the potential for transmission to and from previously partnered men and women who may be seeking new partners at later ages or for the first time in many years (Vance, 2002).

Given these sociological and demographic trends, successful aging with HIV is becoming the next frontier for research, prevention, health maintenance, and social services. Despite attention given to older adults contracting HIV (Moore & Amburgey, 2000), little attention has been focused on how people are aging with the disease (Vance, 2002). Research is required to delineate the multiple biopsychosocial issues that are unique to older adults who are newly infected as well as those who have been aging with it.

The purpose of this paper is to address some of the areas in which aging and HIV are juxtaposed and examine how they may impact individuals who will be aging with this diagnosis. This will highlight some of the challenges people confront as they grow older with this disease. By identifying gaps in the literature, research questions are posited as they relate to successful aging. Will people with HIV be more vulnerable to cognitive declines and depression as they age? Does the interaction of age and HIV represent a barrier to building and maintaining social networks? What are the considerations for those returning to work due to improved health but facing an uncertain retirement? What comorbid medical problems are exacerbated by the combined influence of HIV and aging? Ultimately, what factors are important in understanding how to age successfully with HIV?

DEFINING SUCCESSFUL AGING

The topic of successful aging in the gerontological literature has various definitions, but thus far Kahana and Kahana (2001) appear to be the only authors who deliberately link successful aging with HIV. They proposed the Preventive and Corrective Proactivity Model of Successful Aging. In this complex model (7 main variables, 19 minor variables, 11 paths), the guiding principle asserts that persons, using their own coping and individual dispositions, focus existing resources to confront stressors related to HIV or aging in order to maximize quality of life outcomes. This model considers the interactions between one's disposition for successful aging and one's external resources, although the precise mechanisms of these interactions have yet to be determined empirically. Since only one model exists in this area, alternative models are necessary to stimulate a dialogue in order to conceptualize the many issues that accompany aging with HIV. At the core of all successful aging models must be the notion that to affect the best possible outcome for the person, remaining (or compensatory) psychological, physical, and social resources must be utilized.

Successful aging consists of a number of biopsychosocial elements. Psychological and sociological elements of successful aging include hardiness, active social participation, having many friends, and being satisfied with life. For example, Laferriere and Hamel-Bissell (1994) studied the lives of women over the age of 85 who were defined as "hardy" by their community and found that working hard and staying active, being with family and friends, and consciously dealing with the hard times were all important traits of successful aging. Additionally, emotional concepts such as trust have emerged as predictors of successful aging (Barefoot, Maynard, Beckman, Brummet, Hooker, & Siegler, 1998).

Physical elements of successful aging include participating in health-promoting behaviors, refraining from poor health habits, and remaining physically competent. For example, Avlund, Holstein, Mortensen, and Schroll (1999) found that for men, good self-rated physical health was related to their definition of successful aging. Likewise, Ford et al. (2000) defined successful aging as the ability to remain independent and autonomous; they found that good physical functioning and having fewer chronic conditions predicted successful aging. In a landmark longitudinal study, Valient and Mukamal (2001) followed adolescents for over 60 years and analyzed factors related to successful aging as defined by health, death and disability before age 80, social supports, and mental health. In addition to personal factors such as coping mechanisms, health-related behaviors such as alcohol abuse, smoking, exercise, and body mass index were robust in predicting the quality of successful aging.

Successful aging is a multifactorial concept that can be either general or specific. Baltes and Baltes (1998) broadly defined successful aging, with its components being length of life, biological health, mental health, cognitive efficiency, social competence and productivity, personal control, and life satisfaction. Conversely, Roos and Havens (1991) specifically defined successful aging as being independent in mobility and activities of daily living, exercising cognitive efficiency, and not receiving nursing home or home care services. Although these definitions implicitly incorporate biopsychosocial aspects necessary to define successful aging, Rowe and Kahn (1997) explicitly defined successful aging with psychological, social, and physical domains of aging. A three-pronged definition proposed by Rowe and Kahn includes low probability of disease, high cognitive and functional capacity, and an active engagement with life. Similarly, successful aging in this paper is defined as being cognitively and emotionally functional, having supportive social networks that fulfill personal and intimate needs, and avoiding medical problems while retaining vigor and mobility.

Obviously, to those who are aging "normally" as well as to those aging with HIV, declines in all three areas are inevitable to some degree. As mentioned, successful aging requires compensation, adaptation, and reframing goals when declines occur. In other words, to successfully age one makes do with the remaining abilities and resources one still has. Someone aging with HIV may retire sooner rather than later since statistically one is more likely to experience health problems sooner in life. A person already experiencing health problems that impede mobility and social contact may compensate by finding other ways to socialize such as by using the internet like many infirmed elders do, instead of withdrawing (White et al., 2002). Finally, successful aging does not emphasize halting the aging process; instead, it concentrates on achieving the highest possible quality of life while avoiding negative influences that can deplete personal resources.

FACTORS AFFECTING PERSONS AGING WITH HIV

Despite the biopsychosocial complications of living with HIV, successfully aging with this disease is possible. In fact, studying a large sample, Perez and

Moore (2003) recently observed no significant difference in mortality rates between younger (18-49) and older adults (50+) who received HAART. This demonstrates the efficacy of HIV drug treatment in older adults. The direct pathophysiological consequences of HIV infection and its associated therapies combined with the aging process impact major areas of an individual's life.

Table 1 shows examples of how aging and HIV exert influence and intersect. It is presently uncertain whether the combined influences of both aging and HIV result in detrimental additive, synergistic, or independent effects on function and adaptation. Potential factors affecting both aging and HIV related to psychological, social, and physiological function are now discussed using selected examples.

PSYCHOLOGICAL FUNCTIONING

Psychological components of successful aging include cognitive efficiency, hardiness, and a "can do" attitude. While both aging and HIV can wield a harmful effect on psychological functioning on many different levels, there are at least two possible domains where the psychology of aging and HIV may create negative synergistic effects. First, the combined influence of aging and HIV may result in declines in cognitive functioning, especially psychomotor impairment. Second, their combined influences may create a vulnerability to emotional problems, specifically depression. Obviously, both of these can dramatically impact one's functional status, autonomy, and quality of life (Osowieki et al., 2000).

Age-related cognitive declines are well established phenomena in the aging literature. Gradual mental declines in some areas are accepted as a part of normal aging while sudden severe declines are identified as pathological aging (Schaie, 1996). Specifically, normal changes have been observed in domains of executive functioning (West, 1996), attention (McDowd & Shaw, 2000), memory (Floyd & Scogin, 1997), and speed of processing (Kail & Salthouse, 1994). The likely etiology for these declines is related to age-related neural changes and brain functioning.

Cognitive declines have also been observed with advanced HIV. Prior to the widespread use of HAART, AIDS Dementia Complex (ADC) was more common than currently. The etiological mechanism underlying ADC is believed to center around the direct effect of HIV within the central nervous system, producing neurotoxins that destroy glial cells which promote neuronal health (Stern, 1994). Currently with appropriate antiretroviral treatment, there is contradictory information about whether HIV still causes such declines in cognitive functioning (Grassi et al., 1995; Herning et al., 2000; Suarez et al., 2001). In addition, certain HAART medications have prevalent central nervous system side effects that result in cognitive deficits. For instance, efavirenz (a widely used and highly effective antiretroviral) is known to produce

TABLE 1. Examples of Synthesis of Age-Related and HIV-Related Changes

	Age-Related Changes	Synthesis and Hypotheses	HIV-Related Changes
Psychological: Cognitive	Cortical and subcortical declines in executive functioning, memory, and speed of processing have been observed with age (Schaie, 1996).	Aging with HIV may result in a marked reduction in psychomotor speed.	Subcortical declines in psychomotor speed have been observed with HIV (Christensson et al., 1999).
Psychological: Emotional	Suicide rates for white elderly men are 3.5 times greater than the normal population (Gallagher-Thompson & Osgood, 1997).	Depression may be even higher in adults aging with HIV. Likewise, suicide rates may be even higher for older men with HIV.	Suicide rates for HIV-positive men are 35 times the normal population (Joseph et al., 1990).
Social: Disengagement	Disengagement and feelings of loneliness are common in aging (Fees et al., 1999).	People aging with HIV may be at risk of social disengagement and may experience specific problems related to reintegrating into social environments.	Adults with HIV experiencing the Lazarus Effect are faced with the opportunity to reengage in the process of living (Scott & Constantine, 1999).
Social: Financial	Retirement has become a normal developmental process for many older adults (Gustman & Steinmeier, 2001-2002).	Retirement futures for adults with HIV are compromised due to impaired productivity, job performance, perceived lack of long-term survival, and immediate financial concerns. Thus, the financial future of older adults with HIV is tenuous.	Adults with HIV experience symptoms such as fatigue and depression that may impair productivity, job performance, and job security. In addition, many perceiving that they were not going to be around for the future, or were living from hand-to-mouth, did not prepare for retirement (Brooks & Kosinski, 1999).
Medical: CD4+ Cell Production	CD4+ cell production declines with age (Moore & Amburgey, 2000).	Although viral management will be important, augmenting CD4+ cell production must become a more important consideration.	HIV destroys CD4+ cells and overwhelms the immune system's ability to create CD4+ cells (Ho et al., 1995).
Medical: Mitochondrial Damage	Mitochondrial damage occurs with age, resulting in decreased energy (Cortopassi & Arnheim, 1990).	The combined influence of age and HIV may exacerbate mitochondrial damage that impairs overall health, reduces energy, and decreases quality of life.	Mitochondrial damage occurs due to HIV and HIV-related medication, resulting in decreased energy (Chen et al., 1991).

psychosis in some individuals (Lang, Halleguen, Picard, Lang, & Danion, 2001). HAART has been implicated in the development of hypertension, dyslipidemia, and insulin-resistance, which have been associated with declines in a wide variety of mental abilities (Heath et al., 2001). The long-term effects of these medications coupled with the aging process are unknown.

It is hypothesized that as individuals age with HIV, they may become susceptible to symptoms of parkinsonism with associated mental problems (Kousilieri, Sopper, Scheller, ter Meulen, & Riederer, 2002). This hypothesis is based upon observations that show characteristics of HIV similar to the development of Parkinson's disease and that age itself is also a risk factor. Age-related subcortical changes occur that create tremor and slowed thought processing (Savage, 1997). Similar changes have been observed in HIV patients (Wilkie et al., 2003). Some consensus exists that HIV positive individuals experience declines in psychomotor speed (a subcortical ability) known as Mild Cognitive Motor Impairment (Sacktor et al., 1999; Osowieki et al., 2000). HIV infection has been associated with insults in the basal ganglia and substantia nigra, neuronal structures necessary for psychomotor functioning, initiation and perseveration, and smooth regulated movement (Christensson, Ljungberg, Ryding, Svenson, & Rosen, 1999). Furthermore, subcortical diseases, such as Parkinson's disease, that damage the basal ganglia and cause psychomotor impairment, generally increase in frequency with age (Paulsen et al., 1995). Further evidence comes from anecdotal reports that HIV-positive adults taking neuroleptics and psychostimulants experience parkinsonian-type symptoms (Nath et al., 2000). Such medications create similar side-effects in many elderly persons (Julien, 1998), which reinforces the above hypothesis. With observed cognitive changes in both aging and HIV, aging may exacerbate HIV-related cognitive changes. Since age-related changes occur in both cortical and subcortical structures and HIV-related changes occur predominantly in subcortical structures, the interplay between these has yet to be understood.

In addition to the influence of cognition on well-being, aging and HIV possess similar risk patterns for liability. In fact, depression is observed more often in both groups than in the general population (Honn & Bornstein, 2002; Lyketsos et al., 1993; McIntosh, 1993; Zorrilla, McKay, Lubersky, & Schmidt, 1996). However, the long-term effects of living with a socially stigmatizing disease such as HIV are unknown given the previously short lifespan of individuals with this disease. From this, several questions arise. What coping strategies are effective for individuals who are aging well with this disease? Are individuals more at risk for depression and suicide as they age with HIV? Research indicates that individuals, in general, face many psychological adjustments as they age such as declining physical attractiveness, loss of significant others, declines in productivity, loss of meaningful roles, and changes in lifestyle patterns, all of which can contribute to depression (McIntosh, 1993). The emotional impact of some of these same losses may be compounded for individuals with HIV by unique disease-related losses such as financial stress, non-availability of sex partners, and disease stigmatization. Depending upon one's ability to cope, these factors can dramatically contribute to anxiety and depression. Only as more people age with HIV will we learn which individuals can adjust to these multiple issues and which are more at risk for developing depressive symptoms.

The concept of crisis competence suggests that individuals who successfully traverse a crisis period in their lives are more capable of overcoming new challenges such as aging. For instance, David and Knight (2002) found that older adults who overcame obstacles to accepting their sexual orientation as homosexual were better equipped psychologically to cope with their aging status than their heterosexual counterparts. Nevertheless, one's crisis competence may be overwhelmed by the multiple issues present with aging and HIV. Accompanying this, many live with the idea that their disease, although currently stable, may be uncontrollable or unmanageable at a latter point in time. Believing that death and disability can fall on them at any moment can tax the hardiest of coping strategies–a phenomenon known as Damocles syndrome, taken from the story of Damocles' sword which can fall without warning. This has been observed in cancer patients experiencing remission who live with the constant fear that the cancer will return to claim their life (Zebrack & Zeltzer, 2001). The added uncertainty of the aging process may counteract previous crisis competence, producing psychological vulnerability to normal stressors.

With depression being prevalent in both aging and HIV, suicide is another relevant consideration (Conwell et al., 1996). The risk factors for suicide are high in both the elderly and HIV populations. For instance, older white men over the age of 65 have a suicide rate (43.5 per 100,000) which is 3.5 times greater than the normal population (Gallagher-Thompson & Osgood, 1997). Likewise, HIV-positive men have a suicide rate 35 times that of the general population (Joseph et al., 1990); however, this finding was before the optimism created by HAART. Age and HIV are independent risk factors for suicide, but aging with HIV may place individuals at even greater risk for suicide. Race plays a factor as well. Old African American men are much less likely to commit suicide than older white men (Gallagher-Thompson & Osgood, 1997); therefore, white men aging with HIV may be at particular risk of suicide. Obviously, research is necessary to develop targeted services and interventions to buffer against stress and abate depression in this population.

SOCIAL FUNCTIONING

Social components of successful aging include having a network of social support and financial well-being. Adequate social support improves quality of life and is critical for coping with adverse life events. In fact, the number and quality of social supports can ameliorate depression (DuPertuis, Aldwin, &

Bosse, 2001). Feelings of loneliness increase for many older adults (Fees, Martin, & Poon, 1999). Loneliness has also been observed with advanced HIV as people disengaged from friends and family and prepared to die. For those who benefit from HAART, many have been reawakened to a new life as though they were resurrected–aptly called the Lazarus effect (Scott & Constantine, 1999). Where once individuals living with HIV accepted their impending fate and withdrew from social circles and careers, many are now reemerging into the world–returning to work, reacquainting with old friends, building new social networks, and beginning new lives. Although many have expressed difficulty in reintegrating into the process of living (Scott & Constantine, 1999), this may be especially problematic for older persons who perceive themselves as having less time or less to offer. Chesney, Chambers, Taylor, and Johnson (2003) observed this phenomenon and found that older men with HIV had fewer social supports that detrimentally impacted their level of distress and quality of life. This is unfortunate given that high distress and low social support can accelerate disease progression (Leserman et al., 1999). So, as younger adults with HIV may be capable of reinvesting themselves into new roles, older adults may find themselves starting over while their age-matched peers have moved on with their lives (e.g., having families, owning property, career advancement, community involvement). This can create a great amount of dissonance and regret for some older adults with HIV who feel left out, unable to catch up to where they feel they should be.

Financial issues present another source of social stress for many aging with HIV. Prior to HAART, many individuals experienced diminished capacity to work, requiring federal, state, or private disability pensions or income assistance for an extensive period of time. As health improves, entitlements can be lost, requiring persons to reenter the work force despite being somewhat ill from either HIV-related conditions or medications. Some find themselves unable to perform at comparable levels to their non-infected counterparts (Brooks & Kosinski, 1999). Older HIV-positive individuals who reenter the work force are faced with the fact that their contemporaries are near retirement. With serious financial crises and prior low expectations for long-term survival, many find themselves unprepared for retirement. Furthermore, with out-dated job skills, incomplete work histories, and limited career development due to pressing medical concerns, many are poorly positioned to ever make sufficient incomes to subsequently anticipate a secure retirement. This is especially evident in those who contracted the disease through injection drug use (Crystal et al., 2003).

PHYSIOLOGICAL FUNCTIONING

Physical components of successful aging include being mobile, autonomous, and as disease-free as possible. Having HIV precludes being disease-free, but successful aging with HIV can be augmented by reducing risks for or controlling other diseases and chronic conditions and by engaging in health-related behaviors that promote wellness and autonomy. Aging and HIV combine to create unique health problems that represent some of the most fundamental problems elders will face.

Aging and HIV overlap with several physiological issues. The most conspicuous example concerns immune system dysfunction. The hallmark of HIV disease progression lies in the decline of CD4+ lymphocyte (helper T-cell) numbers, which results in impairments of both humoral and cell-mediated immune response (Ho et al., 1995). These impairments leave an individual with advanced HIV disease unable to combat foreign pathogens such as bacteria, viruses, fungi, and protozoa. Aging is also associated with various cell-mediated and humoral immune impairments (Morley, 1999). Age and HIV-related immune impairments act additively to lessen an individual's defense against opportunistic pathogens.

Cardiovascular disease, of which arteriosclerosis is the leading cause of mortality among older adults in the United States, is quite common and age, per se, is the single highest risk factor for it (Lakatta, 2002). The increasing incidence of cardiovascular disease with age is linked to increases in weight, cholesterol, diabetes, and hypertension (Burke, et al., 2001). Likewise, HIV-positive individuals may be at higher risk for cardiovascular disease because of metabolic abnormalities due to antiretroviral treatment with protease inhibitors or HIV itself. The constellation of metabolic abnormalities, termed lipo-dystrophy syndrome (LDS), includes abdominal fat accumulation, increases in cholesterol and triglyceride levels, and insulin resistance (Carr et al., 1998; Hadigan et al., 1999). Premature arteriosclerosis including infarction and need for revascularization has been associated with LDS and reported in individuals while on HAART (David, Hornung, & Fichtenbaum, 2002; Muise & Arbess, 2001). The logical assumption is that with age individuals with HIV will be at risk for developing cardiovascular disease.

Osteopenia (bone loss) is an accompaniment of aging in all humans. It occurs faster in women than in men and more rapidly in some bones than others (Nordin et al., 1998). With age, many bones become "osteoporotic," putting individuals at higher risk for fractures (Seeman, 2002). Recently, osteopenia has been recognized as a significant consequence of HIV, antiretroviral therapy, or both (Huang, Rietschel, Hadigan, Rosenthal, & Grinspoon, 2001; Lawal, Engelson, Wange, Heymsfield, & Kotter, 2001). Case studies provide evidence that HIV-positive individuals on HAART are at risk for pathological fractures due to significant bone loss (Guaraldi et al., 2001). Accelerated bone loss and risk for fractures may emerge as a significant problem for an aging HIV-positive population.

A final physiological problem related to both aging and HIV is mitochondrial dysfunction. Mitochondria are the cellular organelles that produce all cellular energy and metabolism. As people age, mitochondrial DNA (mtDNA) mutations occur (Cortopassi & Arnheim, 1990), resulting in decreased energy synthesis. In fact, a "mitochondrial theory of aging" has been suggested as the mechanism behind many physiological processes of aging (Ozawa, 1998). It is well established that treatment with the class of antiretrovirals called nucleoside reverse transcriptase inhibitors (or NRTIs) can deplete mtDNA (Chen, Vazquez-Padua, & Cheng, 1991; Medina, Tsai, Hsiung, & Cheng, 1994), resulting in declines of mtDNA-encoded mitochondrial enzymes, thereby altering mitochondrial function. Hence, people aging with HIV may face severe mitochondrial damage due to long-term use of medications, coupled with the normal aging process. If so, this will impair organ function as well as result in chronic fatigue.

INTERACTION OF AGING AND HIV

Prior models of successful aging incorporate the interaction of psychological, social, and physiological domains such that a disruption in one area creates ripples that impact other areas. For instance, a decline in physiological health can impact psychological and social functioning. Such ripples may be more challenging in aging with HIV due to the loss of internal and external resources that can accompany HIV. To illustrate how such an interaction can occur, mitochondrial damage will be used to demonstrate how a physiological phenomenon can lead to a host of other problems that diminish an individual's quality of life.

Figure 1 illustrates the interaction of the three major domains of successful aging. Starting with the physiological domain in path A, mitochondrial damage can produce fatigue which impacts psychological functioning, such as causing depression and suppressing cognitive abilities (Corless et al., 2000; Keene et al., 2001; Millikin, Rourke, Halman, & Power, 2003). In path B, declines in cognitive ability and reduced mood can precipitate social isolation (Roberts, Kaplan, Shema, & Strawbridge, 1997). In path C, fatigue can also contribute to reductions in social contact and productivity (Harpham, 1999). In path D, social withdrawal could prevent one from remaining active or having any sort of accountability (e.g., a work out buddy), even though general activity and physical exercise could mitigate some of the detrimental effects and symptoms of fatigue (McAuley et al., 2000). In path E, declines in social interaction may further contribute to depression (DuPertuis, Aldwin, & Bosse, 2001), which in itself can produce a negative feedback loop that perpetuates this condition. In path F, depression and declines in cognitive functioning may prevent self-monitoring behavior from occurring properly, thus reducing health-promoting behaviors such as medication adherence, proper nutrition, and exercise (Wahlqvist & Saviage, 2000). Clearly, when considered through a biopsychosocial model, methods for aging successfully with HIV must be devised in order to reverse the destructive cycle that can occur.

FIGURE 1. The Effects of Age-Related and HIV-Related Mitochondrial Damage on Quality of Life

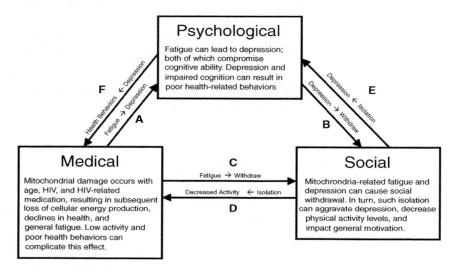

POTENTIAL INTERVENTIONS TO FACILITATE SUCCESSFUL AGING

Social work has the flexibility to intervene in several areas that can significantly improve the internal and external resources that contribute to the process of successful aging. Whether this flexibility resides in counseling, disseminating information and educating, connecting adults to community programs or external resources, or advocacy, a variety of areas must be targeted for intervention in older HIV-positive adults. For instance, interventions and services need to be developed to help older adults with HIV reenter the workforce, create aggressive retirement plans to compensate for years of lost income, confront depression, and assuage stigma related to HIV and ageism (Coon, Lipman, & Ory, 2003). Interventions are especially relevant for HIV-positive individuals as they develop symptoms, the emergence of which is often accompanied by anxiety, dysphoria, and fear. This becomes particularly important when such stressors and the uncertainties about HIV are compounded by age-related declines.

Effective interventions for this dually affected population should be multidisciplinary. For instance, since successful aging depends on the interaction of biopsychosocial factors, several biobehavioral interventions have already been developed with HIV-positive samples (for a comprehensive review see

Robinson and colleagues) (Robinson, Mathews, & Witek-Janusek, 2000). In general, cognitive behavioral stress management (Lutgendorf et al., 1997) and aerobic exercise (Bopp, Phillips, Fulk, & Hand, 2003; Smith et al., 2001) had significant positive effects on psychological and physiological parameters in HIV disease, such as decreased depression and improved health including increasing CD4+ lymphocyte counts. Connecting individuals to both of these interventions could be combined and modified to incorporate coping skills focusing on specific age-related problems, such as changes in personal appearance or declines in energy, to develop comprehensive interventions for adults aging with HIV.

Three primary age-related topics require special attention to help older adults with HIV age successfully: financial/retirement planning, social isolation, and sex education. As mentioned previously, financial matters are a major stress for older adults with HIV since retirement options are limited (Crystal et al., 2003). They need guidance to financial planners, education on retirement options, and linkages to existing programs to supplement existing incomes. In some cases this means retooling and reentering the workforce; for others with poorer health, finding flexible part-time work opportunities or state-supported retirement may be necessary. In either case, social workers can help by providing clients aging with HIV the means to find financial services, retirement programs, or flexible work that meets their particular needs.

Social support has been documented as more important in mitigating distress and augmenting well-being in older men with HIV than in a younger cohort (Chesney et al., 2003). Social support interventions that seek to improve contact and form relationships must be sought. Support groups, care teams, and religious organizations are a good start in the formation of such supports. Unfortunately, internalized HIV-related stigma or even perceptions of one's own aging may hinder the social efforts of many older adults. In such cases, counseling, re-education about HIV and/or aging, and social skills training may be useful. Such interventions may prove helpful in forming natural social supports or even intimate relationships. Social workers must endeavor to recognize social isolation in this population and introduce their clients to organizations and programs that will promote personal contact and social interaction.

Avoiding disease is an essential component of successful aging. The older population who contracted HIV via sexual transmission must avoid reinfection or infection from other sexually transmitted diseases such as hepatitis (Coleman, 2003). Safer sex interventions and other efforts aimed at changing sexual conduct in older men and women must be carefully crafted and age sensitive. Advertisements and flyers must depict older people instead of younger adults. Porsche and Swayser (2003) describe a variety of HIV prevention interventions that can be adapted to older adults such as AIDS risk reduction education, safer sex house parties, sexual assertiveness training, self-management skills, individual risk reduction plans, and HIV prevention case management. Social workers should acknowledge the potential for reinfection in this group and provide the necessary sex education or programming in order to help their clients remain as healthy as possible.

As Coon and colleagues (2003) have pointed out in great detail, any intervention that targets the aging HIV population must do so with several considerations. First, behavioral change occurs within a larger cultural context; interventions must be built from within the culture, not imposed from outside. Second, practitioners must understand how behavioral change actually occurs in order to develop a plan. Third, behavior should be viewed as a moving target, dependent on the vacillations of sociocultural and personal influences. Fourth, healthy behaviors are dependent upon the adoption and maintenance of skills that are generalizable to multiple sociocultural contexts. Fifth, healthy behaviors are maintained by follow-up training or booster sessions. Finally, sustained behavioral change in the person depends on a variety of techniques that target the issue from one or a combination of approaches.

CONCLUSIONS AND FUTURE DIRECTIONS

Successful aging involves the incorporation of health-promoting behaviors and the elimination of harmful behaviors in order to maximize one's quality of life. For example, of the most common types of cancer associated with aging, only lung cancer is found proportionately higher in HIV infection; however, this effect most likely reflects the high prevalence of heavy smoking among HIV-positive adults (Engels, 2001). Thus, behavior is an essential component of the biopsychosocial model of successful aging.

Multiple challenges face individuals aging with HIV and their care providers. Research is needed in order to expand understanding on this new phenomenon. To do so, theoretical models that incorporate aspects of successful aging must be created to help guide such research. In conducting the research, several major caveats must be addressed. First, research will be obfuscated by the many confounding factors that influence HIV prognosis and successful aging such as recreational drug use, reinfection, medication adherence, drug resistance, iatrogenic effects of medications, temperament, hardiness, and spirituality. Second, defining who is "older" will be a consideration (Levy, Holmes, & Smith, 2003). Third, determining which subset of older adults to study must be chosen (Levy et al., 2003). For example, how is life different for those newly diagnosed compared to those who have been HIV-positive for many years? What characteristics differentiate long-term survivors from short-term survivors? How is the aging process different for people who contracted HIV either by blood transfusion, sexual contact, or IV drug use? What long-term effects of medication might now be prevented?

In addition, gender, race, and cultural factors will undoubtedly be important determinants for how people age with HIV (Montoya & Whitsett, 2003).

How age and race interact with HIV is yet to be understood; however, distinct ethnic-oriented coping strategies must be considered in the development of interventions and services. Finally, for the infected person, the processes of aging and disease are inextricable, such that the causes of symptoms and changes are difficult to determine. For example, "Am I tired because I'm HIV-positive or because I'm getting older?" Today such questions challenge clinicians unsure of how to respond to problems that arise. In emerging gerontology and HIV research, there are more questions than answers. As the HIV population ages, finding answers to these questions will grow in importance for those living with HIV and those providing assistance and direction to them.

REFERENCES

Avlund, K., Holstein, B. E., Mortensen, E. L., & Schroll, M. (1999). Active life in old age: Combining measures of functional ability and social participation. *Danish Medical Bulletin*, 46(4), 345-349.

Baltes, P. B. & Baltes, M. M. (1998). *Successful aging: Perspectives from the behavioral sciences*. Cambridge, England: Cambridge University Press.

Barefoot, J. C., Maynard, K. E., Beckman, J. C., Brummet, B. H., Hooker, K., & Siegler, I. C. (1998). Trust, health, and longevity. *Journal of Behavioral Medicine*, 21(6), 517-526.

Bopp, C. M., Phillips, K. D., Fulk, L. J., & Hand, G. A. (2003). Clinical implications of therapeutic exercises in HIV/AIDS. *Journal of the Association of Nurses in AIDS Care*, 14(1), 73-78.

Brooks, R. A., & Kosinski, L. E. (1999). Assisting person living with HIV/AIDS to return to work: Programmatic steps for AIDS service organizations. *AIDS Education and Prevention*, 11(3), 212-223.

Burke, G. L., Arnold, A. M., Bild, D. E., Cushman, M., Fried, L. P., Newman, A. et al. (2001). Factors associated with healthy aging: The cardiovascular health study. *Journal of the American Geriatrics Society*, 49(3), 254-262.

Carr, A., Samaras, K., Burton, S., Law, M., Freund, J., Chisholm, D. J. et al. (1998). A syndrome of peripheral lipodystrophy, hyperlipidaemia and insulin resistance in patients receiving HIV protease inhibitors. *AIDS*, 12(7), F51-58.

Chen, C. H., Vazquez-Padua, M., & Cheng, Y. C. (1991). Effect of anti-human immunodeficiency virus nucleoside analogs on mitochondrial DNA and its implication for delayed toxicity. *Molecular Pharmacology*, 39(5), 625-8.

Chesney, M. A., Chambers, D. B., Taylor, J. M., & Johnson, L. M. (2003). Social support, distress, and well-being in older men living with HIV infection. *JAIDS Journal of Acquired Immune Deficiency Syndrome*, 33, S185-S193.

Christensson, B., Ljungberg, B., Ryding, E., Svenson, G., & Rosen, I. (1999). SPECT with 99mTc-HMPAO in subjects with HIV infections: Cognitive dysfunction correlates with high uptake. *Scandinavian Journal of Infectious Disease*, 31, 349-354.

Coleman, C. L. (2003). Transmission of HIV infection among older adults: A population at risk. *Journal of the Association of Nurses in AIDS Care*, 14(1), 82-85.

Conwell, Y., Duberstein, P. R., Cox, C., Herrmann, J. H., Forbes, N. T., & Caine, E. D. (1996). Relationships of age and Axis I diagnoses in victims of completed suicide: A psychological autopsy study. *American Journal of Psychiatry*, 153, 1001-1008.

Coon, D. W., Lipman, P. D., & Ory, M. G. (2003). Designing effective HIV/AIDS social and behavioral interventions for the population of those age 50 and older. *JAIDS Journal of Acquired Immune Syndromes*, 33, S194-S205.

Corless, I. B., Bakken, S., Nicholas, P. K., Holzemer, W. L., McGibbon, C. A., Inouye, J. et al. (2000). Predictors of perception of cognitive functioning in HIV/AIDS. *Journal of the Association of Nurses in AIDS Care*, 11(3), 19-26.

Cortopassi, G. A. & Arnheim, N. (1990). Detection of a specific mitochondrial DNA deletion in tissues of older humans. *Nucleic Acids Research*, 18(23), 6927-6933.

Crystal, S., Akincigil, A., Sambamoorthi, U., Wenger, N., Fleishman, J. A., Zingmond, D. S. et al. (2003). The diverse older HIV-positive population: A national profile of economic circumstances, social support, and quality of life. *JAIDS Journal of Acquired Immune Deficiency Syndromes*, 33, S76-S83.

David, M. H., Hornung, R., & Fichtenbaum, C. J. (2002). Ischemic cardiovascular disease in persons with human immunodeficiency virus infection. *Clinical Infectious Diseases*, 34(1), 98-102.

David, S., & Knight, B. (2002). *Stress and coping among lesbian, gay, bisexual, and transgender older adults*. Presentation at the American Psychological Association annual meeting.

DuPertuis, L. L., Aldwin, C. M., & Bosse, R. (2001). Does the source of support matter for different health outcomes? *Journal of Aging and Health*, 13(4), 494-510.

Engels, E. A. (2001). Human immunodeficiency virus infection, aging, and cancer. *Journal of Clinical Epidemiology*, 54, S29-S34.

Fees, B. S., Martin, P., & Poon, L. W. (1999). A model of loneliness in older adults. *Journals of Gerontology*, 54(4), P231-P239.

Floyd, M. & Scogin, F. (1997). Effects of memory training on the subjective memory functioning and mental health of older adults: A meta-analysis. *Psychology and Aging* 12(1), 150-161.

Ford, A. B., Haug, M. R., Stange, K. C., Gaines, A. D., Noelker, L. S., & Jones, P. K. (2000). Sustained personal autonomy: A measure of successful aging. *Journal of Aging and Health*, 12(4), 470-489.

Gallagher-Thompson, D. & Osgood, N. J. (1997). Suicide in later life. *Behavior Therapy* 28, 23-41.

Grassi, M. P., Clerici, F., Perin, C., Zocchetti, C., Borella, M., Cargnel, A. et al. (1995). HIV infection and drug use: Influence on cognitive function. *AIDS*, 9(2), 165-170.

Guaraldi, G., Ventura, P., Albuzza, M., Orlando, G., Bedini, A., Amorico, G., & Esposito, R. (2001). Pathological fractures in AIDS patients with osteopenia and osteoporosis induced by antiretroviral therapy. *AIDS*, 15(1), 137-138.

Gustman, A. L., & Steinmeier, T. L. (2001-2002). Retirement and wealth. *Social Security Bulletin*, 64(2), 66-91.

Hadigan, C., Miller, K., Corcoran, C., Anderson, E., Basgoz, N., & Grinspoon, S. (1999). Fasting hyperinsulinemia and changes in regional body composition in human immunodeficiency virus-infected women. *Journal of Clinical Endocrinology & Metabolism*, 84(6), 1932-1937.

Harpham, W. S. (1999). Resolving the frustration of fatigue. *Cancer Journal for Clinicians*, 49(3), 178-189.

Heath, K. V., Hogg, R. S., Chan, K. J., Harris, M., Montessori, V., O'Shaughnessy, M. V., & Montanera, J. S. (2001). Lipodystrophy-associated morphological, cholesterol and triglyceride abnormalities in a population-based HIV/AIDS treatment database. *AIDS*, 15(2), 231-239.

Herning, R. I., Better, W. E., Nelson, R., Corelick, D., & Cadet, J. L. (2000). Antiviral medications improve cerebrovascular perfusion in HIV+ non-drug users and HIV+ cocaine abusers. *Annals of the New York Academy of Sciences*, 890, 405-412.

Ho, D. D., Neumann, A. U., Perelson, A. S., Chen, W., Leonard, J. M., & Markowitz, M. (1995). Rapid turnover of plasma virions and CD4 lymphocytes in HIV-1 infection. *Nature*, 373(6510), 123-126.

Honn, V. J. & Bornstein, R. A. (2002). Social support, neuropsychological performance, and depression in HIV infection. *Journal of the International Neuropsychological Society*, 8, 436-447.

Huang, J. S., Rietschel, P., Hadigan, C. M., Rosenthal, D. I., & Grinspoon, S. (2001). Increased abdominal visceral fat is associated with reduced bone density in HIV-infected men with lipodystrophy. *AIDS*, 15(8), 975-82.

Joseph, J. G., Caumartin, S. M., Tal., M., Kirscht, J. P., Kessler, R. C., Ostrow, D. G. et al. (1990). Psychological functioning in a cohort of gay men at risk for AIDS: A three-year descriptive study. *Journal of Nervous and Mental Disorders*, 178, 607-615.

Julien, R. M. (1998). *A primer of drug action*. New York: W. H. Freeman.

Kahana, E., & Kahana, B. (2001). Successful aging among people with HIV/AIDS. *Journal of Clinical Epidemiology*, 54, S53-S56.

Kail, R. & Salthouse, T. A. (1994). Processing speed as a mental capacity. *Acta Psychologica*, 86, 199-225.

Keene, C. D., Rodrigues, C. M., Eich, T., Linehan-Stieers, C., Abt, A., Kren, B. T. et al. (2001). A bile acid protects against motor and cognitive deficits and reduces striatal degeneration in the 3-nitropropionic acid model of Huntington's disease. *Experimental Neurology*, 171(2), 351-360.

Koutsilieri, E., Sopper, S., Scheller, C., ter Meulen, V., & Riederer, P. (2002). Parkinsonism in HIV dementia. *Journal of Neural Transmission*, 109(5-6), 767-775.

Laferriere, R. H. & Hamel-Bissell, B. P. (1994). Successful aging of oldest old women in the northeast kingdom of Vermont. *IMAGE: Journal of Nursing Scholarship*, 26(4), 319-323.

Lakatta, E. G. (2002). Age-associated cardiovascular changes in health: Impact on cardiovascular disease in older persons. *Heart Failure Reviews*, 7(1), 29-49.

Lang, J. P., Halleguen, O., Picard, A., Lang, J. M., & Danion, J. M. (2001). Apropos of atypical melancholia with Sustiva (efavirenz). *Encephale*, 27(3), 290-3.

Lawal, A., Engelson, E. S., Wange, J., Heymsfield, S. B., & Kotler, D. P. (2001). Equivalent osteopenia in HIV-positive individuals studied before and during the era of highly active antiretroviral therapy. *AIDS*, 15(2), 278-80.

Leserman, J., Jackson, E. D., Petitto, J. M., Golden, R. N., Silva, S. G., Perkins, D. O. et al. (1999). Progression to AIDS: The effects of stress, depressive symptoms, and social support. *Psychosomatic Medicine*, 61, 397-406.

Levy, J. A., Holmes, D., & Smith, M. (2003). Conceptual and methodological issues in research on age and aging. *JAIDS Journal of Acquired Immune Deficiency Syndromes*, 33, S206-S217.

Linsk, N. L. (2000). HIV among old adults: Age-specific issues in prevention and treatment. *AIDS Reader*, 10(7), 430-441.

Lutgendorf, S. K., Antoni, M. H., Irons, G., Starr, K., Costello, N., Zuckerman, M. et al. (1997). Cognitive-behavioral stress management decreases dysphoric mood and herpes simplex virus-type 2 antibody titers in symptomatic HIV-seropositive gay men. *Journal of Consulting & Clinical Psychology* 65(1), 31-43.

Lyketsos, C. G., Hoover, D. R., Guccione, M., Senterfitt, W., Dew, M. A., Wesch, J. et al. (1993). Depressive symptoms as predictors of medical outcomes in HIV infection. *Journal of the American Medical Association*, 270, 2563-2567.

McAuley, E., Blissmer, B., Marquez, D. X., Jerome, G. J., Kramer, A. F., & Katula, J. (2000). Social relations, physical activity, and well-being in older adults. *Preventive Medicine*, 31(5), 608-617.

McDowd, J. M. & Shaw, R. J. (2000). Attention and aging: A functional perspective. In F. I. M. Salthouse (Ed.), *The handbook of aging and cognition*. Mahwah, NJ: Lawrence Erlbaum Associates.

McIntosh, J. L. (1993). Older adults: The next suicide epidemic? *Suicide and Life-Threatening Behavior*, 22(3), 322-332.

Medina, D. J., Tsai, C. H., Hsiung, G. D., & Cheng, Y. C. (1994). Comparison of mitochondrial morphology, mitochondrial DNA content, and cell viability in cultured cells treated with three anti-human immunodeficiency virus dideoxynucleosides. *Antimicrobial Agents & Chemotherapy*, 38(8), 1824-1828.

Millikin, C. P., Rourke, S. B., Halman, M. H., & Power, C. (2003). Fatigue in HIV/AIDS is associated with depression and subjective neurocognitive complaints but not neuropsychological functioning. *Journal of Clinical & Experimental Neuropsychology*, 25(2), 201-215.

Montoya, I. D., & Whitsett, D. D. (2003). New frontiers and challenges in HIV research among older minority populations. *JAIDS Journal of Acquired Immune Deficiency Syndromes*, 33, S218-S221.

Moore, L. W. & Amburgey, L. B. (2000). Older adults with HIV. *AJORN Journal*, 71(4), 873-876.

Morley, J. (1999). Immunosenescence. In R. Coe (Ed.), *Geriatric Science*. Baltimore: Johns Hopkins Press.

Muise, A. & Arbess, G. (2001). The risk of myocardial infarction in HIV-positive patients receiving HAART: A case report. *International Journal of STD & AIDS*, 12(9), 612-613.

Nath, A., Anderson, C., Jones, M., Maragos, W., Booze, R., Mactutus, C., Bell, J. et al. (2000). Neurotoxicity and dysfunction of dopaminergic systems associated with AIDS dementia. *Journal of Psychopharmacology*, 14, 222-227.

Nordin, B. E., Need, A. G., Steurer, T., Morris, H. A., Chatterton, B. E., & Horowitz, M. (1998). Nutrition, osteoporosis, and aging. *Annals of the New York Academy of Sciences*, 854, 336-351.

Osowieki, D. A., Cohen, R. A., Morrow, K. M., Paul, R. H., Carpenter, C. C. J., Flanigan, T. et al. (2000). Neurocognitive and psychological contributions to quality of life in HIV-1 infected women. *AIDS*, 14, 1327-1332.

Ozawa, T. (1998). Mitochondrial DNA mutations and age. *Annals of the New York Academy of Sciences*, 854, 128-54.

Palella, F. J., Delaney, K. M., Moorman, A. C., Loveless, M. O., Fuhrer, J., Satten, G. A. et al. (1998). Declining morbidity and mortality among patients with advanced human immunodeficiency virus infection. HIV Outpatient Study Investigators. *New England Journal of Medicine*, 338(13), 853-860.

Paulsen, J. S., Butters, N., Sadek, B. S., Johnson, S. A., Salmon, D. P., Swerdlow, N. R. et al. (1995). Distinct cognitive profiles of cortical and subcortical dementia in advanced illness. *Neurology*, 45, 951-956.

Perez, J. L., & Moore, R. D. (2003). Greater effect of Highly Active Antiretroviral Therapy on survival in people aged $\geq$ 50 years compared with younger people in an urban observational cohort. *Clinical Infectious Diseases*, 36, 212-218.

Porche, D. J., & Swayzer, R. (2003). HIV prevention: A review of interventions. *Journal of the Association of Nurses in AIDS Care*, 14(1), 79-81.

Roberts, R. E., Kaplan, G. A., Shema, S. J., & Strawbridge, W. J. (1997). Does growing older increase the risk for depression? *American Journal of Psychiatry*, 154(10), 1283-1390.

Robinson, F. P., Mathews, H. L., & Witek-Janusek, L. (2000). Stress reduction and HIV disease: A review of intervention studies using a psychoneuroimmunology framework. *Journal of the Association of Nurses in AIDS Care*, *11*(2), 87-96.

Roos, N. P. & Havens, B. (1991). Predictors of successful aging: A twelve-year study of Manitoba elderly. *American Journal of Public Health*, 81, 63-68.

Rowe, J. W. & Kahn, R. L. (1997). Successful aging. *The Gerontologist*, 37, 433-440.

Sacktor, N. C., Lyles, R. H., Skolasky, R. L., Anderson, D. E., McArthur, J. C., McFarlane, G. et al. (1999). Combination antiretroviral therapy improves psychomotor speed performance in HIV-seropositive homosexual men. *Neurology*, 52, 1640-1647.

Savage, C. R. (1997). Neuropsychology of subcortical dementias. *The Psychiatric Clinics of North America*, *20*(4), 911-931.

Schaie, K. W. (1996). *Intellectual development in adults: The Seattle Longitudinal Study*. New York: Cambridge University Press.

Scott, S., & Constantine, L. M. (1999). The Lazarus syndrome: A second chance for life with HIV infection. *Journal of the American Pharmaceutical Association*, 39(4), 462-466.

Seeman, E. (2002). Pathogensis of bone fragility in women and men. *Lancet*, 359(93-20), 1841-1850.

Slusher, M. P., Halman, L. J., Eshleman, S., & Ostrow, D. (1994). *Patterns of sexual behavior among younger and older gay men*. Presentation at the Gerontological Society of America annual meeting.

Smith, B. A., Neidig, J. L., Nickel, J. T., Mitchell, G. L., Para, M. F., & Fass, R. J. (2001). Aerobic exercise: Effects on parameters related to fatigue, dyspnea, weight and body composition in HIV-positive adults. *AIDS*, 15(6), 693-701.

Stern, R. (1994). Neuropsychiatric aspects of HIV, with a note on psychoneroimmunology. *Advances: Journal of the Institute for the Advancement of Health*, 10(4), 28-31.

Suarez, S., Baril, L., Stankoff, B., Khellaf, M., Dubois, B., Lubetzki, C. et al. (2001). Outcome of patients with HIV-1-related cognitive impairment on highly active antiretroviral therapy. *AIDS*, 15, 195-200.

Tashima, K. T., & Carpenter, C. C. (2003). Fusion inhibitors–a major but costly step forward in the treatment of HIV-1. *New England Journal of Medicine,* 348(22), 2249-2250.

Vaillant, G. E. & Mukamal, K. (2001). Successful aging. *American Journal of Psychiatry,* 158, 839-847.

Vance, D. E. (2002). *Aging successfully with HIV.* Presentation at the American Society on Aging annual meeting.

Wahlqvist, M. L., & Saviage, G. S. (2000). Interventions aimed at dietary and lifestyle changes to promote healthy aging. *European Journal of Clinical Nutrition,* 54, S148-S156.

West, R. L. (1996). An application of prefrontal cortex function theory to cognitive aging. *Psychological Bulletin,* 120, 488-507.

White, H., McConnell, E., Clipp, E., Branch, L. G., Sloane, R., Pieper, C. et al. (2002). A randomized controlled trial of the psychosocial impact of providing internet training and access to older adults. *Aging & Mental Health,* 6(3), 213-221.

Wilkie, F. L., Goodkin, K., Khamis, I., van Zuilen, M. H., Lee, D., Lecusay, R., Concha, M., Symes, S., Suarez, P., & Eisdorfer, C. (2003). Cognitive functioning in younger and older HIV-1-infected adults. *JAIDS Journal of Acquired Immune Deficiency Syndrome,* 33, S93-S105.

Zebrack, B. J., & Zeltzer, L. K. (2001). Living beyond the sword of Damocles: Surviving childhood cancer. *Expert Review of Anticancer Therapy,* 1(2), 163-164.

Zorrilla, E. P., McKay, J. R., Luborsky, L., & Schmidt, K. (1996). Relation of stressors and depressive symptoms to clinical progression of viral illness. *American Journal of Psychiatry,* 153, 626-635.

BRIDGING RESEARCH AND PRACTICE

Compensating for Cognitive Deficits in Persons Aged 50 and Over with HIV/AIDS: A Pilot Study of a Cognitive Intervention

M. M. Neundorfer, PhD, RN
C. J. Camp, PhD
M. M. Lee, PhD
M. J. Skrajner, MA
M. L. Malone, MA
J. R. Carr, MA

SUMMARY. This pilot study describes a cognitive intervention designed to compensate for cognitive deficits among persons with HIV/

M. M. Neundorfer, PhD, RN, is a Research Scientist at Myers Research Institute, Menorah Park Center for Senior Living, 27100 Cedar Road, Beachwood, OH 44122 (E-mail: mneundorfer@myersri.com).

C. J. Camp, PhD, is a Senior Research Scientist and Director of the Myers Research Institute.

M. M. Lee, PhD, is a Post-doctoral Fellow in Psychology at the Veterans' Administration Pittsburgh Health Care System, Pittsburgh, OH.

M. J. Skrajner, MA, is a Research Associate at Myers Research Institute.

M. L. Malone, MA, is a Speech Language Pathologist and Research Associate at Myers Research Institute.

J. R. Carr, MA, is a Speech Therapist at Myers Research Institute.

This research was supported by a grant from the National Institute of Aging, RO3 AG19016, Principal Investigator, C. J. Camp.

[Haworth co-indexing entry note]: "Compensating for Cognitive Deficits in Persons Aged 50 and Over with HIV/AIDS: A Pilot Study of a Cognitive Intervention." Neundorfer et al. Co-published simultaneously in *Journal of HIV/AIDS & Social Services* (The Haworth Press) Vol. 3, No. 1, 2004, pp. 79-97; and: *Midlife and Older Adults and HIV: Implications for Social Service Research, Practice, and Policy* (ed: Cynthia Cannon Poindexter and Sharon M. Keigher) The Haworth Press, Inc., 2004, pp. 79-97. Single or multiple copies of this article are available for a fee from The Haworth Document Delivery Service [1-800-HAWORTH, 9:00 a.m. - 5:00 p.m. (EST). E-mail address: docdelivery@haworthpress.com].

Digital Object Identifier: 10.1300/J187v03n01_07

AIDS aged 50 and over. Seventeen participants were screened for memory and executive function deficits. Ten participants received the intervention, based on Spaced Retrieval (SR) and use of external memory aids. At two months post-treatment, all participants reported that the intervention helped them meet two self-selected functional goals (e.g., remembering to take medications, remembering clinic appointments) and the majority successfully learned and retained the correct memory strategy. Spaced Retrieval, coupled with external aids, has potential for helping persons with HIV adhere to treatment regimens. *[Article copies available for a fee from The Haworth Document Delivery Service: 1-800-HAWORTH. E-mail address: <docdelivery@haworthpress.com> Website: <http://www.Haworth Press.com> © 2004 by The Haworth Press, Inc. All rights reserved.]*

KEYWORDS. HIV, AIDS, older persons, HIV-1 associated cognitive-motor disorders, HAD, dementia, Spaced Retrieval, interventions

Persons aged 50 and over represent fifteen percent of all AIDS cases diagnosed in the United States (CDC, 2003). The number of persons aged 50 and older who are living with HIV/AIDS continues to rise because persons with HIV/AIDS are living longer on current anti-retroviral medications and the number of new infections in this age group is increasing (Ory & Mack, 1998). These individuals are considered "older persons" within the HIV/AIDS demographics, and are also defined as older adults with HIV/AIDS by the National Institute on Aging. They present unique challenges to HIV/AIDS health service professionals. There is evidence that these older persons are likely to have a more rapid progression from HIV infection to AIDS, accelerated progression of AIDS opportunistic illnesses, more complex co-morbid illnesses, longer histories of drug and alcohol abuse and/or mental illness, and fewer community support services than younger persons (Emlet & Farkas, 2001; Heckman et al., 2000; Linsk, 2000; Mack & Bland, 1999). In addition, cognitive deficits associated with HIV/AIDS may be more severe and progress more quickly in older persons with HIV (Goodkin et al., 2001). It is critical that social workers and others providing case management for older persons with HIV/AIDS recognize and address these cognitive deficits because they threaten the ability of persons with HIV/AIDS to manage their illness independently.

Cognitive deficits in those aged 50 and over living with HIV/AIDS, however, have been little studied and interventions to help older persons compensate for these deficits have rarely been tested. This pilot study was designed to (1) identify specific types of cognitive deficits in a small sample of persons aged 50 and over living with HIV/AIDS and (2) demonstrate the potential effectiveness of a cognitive intervention designed to help these persons better manage their complex care regimens.

Multiple neurological conditions are associated with HIV/AIDS, but those most likely to be affected by age are what have been called HIV-1-associated cognitive-motor disorders (Goodkin et al., 2001). HIV-1-associated cognitive-motor disorders may vary from a mild, subclinical change to a clinical disorder of mild severity (minor cognitive-motor disorder or MCMD) on to a dementing illness (HIV-1 associated dementia or HAD) that involves impairment in cognitive, behavioral, and/or motor spheres. It is estimated that one-third of the adult HIV+ population develops HAD (Koutsilieri, ter Meulen, & Riederer, 2001). Although research findings are mixed with regard to whether persons who are HIV+ exhibit significant cognitive deficits prior to developing AIDS, White et al. (1995) concluded from a review of over 50 studies that asymptomatic HIV+ individuals were about three times more likely to show neuropsychological deficits than their counterparts without HIV.

Persons with MCMD and HAD initially complain of mild cognitive decline, including difficulty concentrating, remembering things, and completing tasks; in addition, social withdrawal, apathy, irritability, depressed affect and decreased interest in activities are common (Castellon, Hinkin, & Myers, 2000; Goldenberg & Boyle, 2000). These deficits translate into inability to follow directions, problems with keeping appointments, confusion and disorientation, and non-adherence to medications. This pattern of symptoms is consistent with subcortical involvement with projections to the frontal lobe (Castellon et al.; Goodkin et al., 2001). These symptoms are often associated with deficits in executive functioning, a term that has been used to describe higher order cognitive processes that control and integrate other mental activities, including planning/anticipating, organizing, inhibiting irrelevant information, memory (e.g., recall and recognition), judgment and self-monitoring (Bryan & Luszcz, 2000; Ferrer-Caja, Crawford, & Bryan, 2002).

In this study, we chose to focus on executive functioning because: (1) the earliest signs and symptoms of cognitive deficits in HIV are often associated with executive dysfunction. These signs and symptoms can occur in the absence of dementia and yet can still impact critical health behaviors such as medication adherence. (2) problems with executive dysfunction may be especially relevant in older adults with HIV, even if AIDS has not been diagnosed, because declines in executive function are typically seen in healthy older adults compared to younger controls (Ferrer-Caja, Crawford, & Bryan, 2002; Libon et al., 1994; Salthouse, Fristoe, & Rhee, 1996; Winocur, Moscovitch, & Stuss, 1996). In addition, when one considers the likelihood of common comorbid illnesses of older persons, such as cardiovascular disease and strokes, the older person with HIV/AIDS, is at high risk for a wide range of cognitive deficits, including executive dysfunction. (3) a history of substance abuse further threatens cognitive function in persons with HIV/AIDS (Bartok et al., 1997; Martin, Pitrak, Robertson et al., 1995; Martin, Pitrak, Pursell, Mullan, & Novak, 1995; Martin et al., 2003; Taylor et al., 2000). Specifically, a combination of stimulant dependence and HIV produce additive effects for tasks requiring complex decision making and focused attention, resulting from impaired frontal lobe functioning, the primary locus for executive function. It may be likely, therefore, that presence of HIV in older populations could produce effects incremental to those of both normal and pathological aging with respect to impairment in executive functioning.

Clearly, the cognitive deficits, especially executive function deficits, associated with HIV/AIDS and other co-morbidities threaten older persons' abilities to manage HIV/AIDS treatment regimes, including remembering to take multiple doses of medications a day, monitoring symptoms and side effects of the illness as well as the medications, self-reporting adherence to medication regimens, keeping track of multiple medical and other appointments, using feedback to change behavior when medications or appointments are missed, and applying for various types of assistance and support. Therefore, it is critical that health service professionals recognize these cognitive deficits in their clients with HIV/AIDS, especially their older clients, be aware of the impact these deficits have on clients' abilities to adhere to medications, keep appointments, and follow up on recommendations for service, and develop strategies that will help these clients compensate for such deficits.

This study was designed to (1) determine the prevalence of executive dysfunction and other cognitive deficits in our sample, and (2) demonstrate the potential benefit of Spaced Retrieval (SR), coupled with use of external aids to memory, for persons with HIV/AIDS, aged 50 and over, who have executive dysfunction alone or in combination with other cognitive deficits. External aids used in the project included pill organizers, timers, calendars, checklists, and cue cards. SR is a cognitive intervention that helps individuals recall information over clinically meaningful time frames (days, weeks, months). In SR, individuals practice learning and successfully recalling new information over progressively longer time intervals. For example, the participant may be asked, "What do you do after you take your medications?" He/she then tries to recall the response, "Check them off the checklist," at progressively longer time intervals, beginning with 30 seconds and then doubling in length (1 min, 2 min, up to 16 min) on successive trials as information is correctly recalled. If the participant fails to recall the response correctly, the therapist tells the participant the response, asks him/her to repeat it, and reduces the next interval length to the length of the last one at which retrieval was successful. Along with giving the correct response, participants practice executing the strategy (e.g., checking the medications off the checklist). Each session ends with the participant having successfully recalled the response and demonstrated the correct strategy. When the participant is able to recall the correct response and demonstrate the correct strategy at the start of three consecutive training sessions (each spaced 2-5 days apart), then the participant has achieved "initial mastery." In essence, SR is a shaping paradigm applied to memory, with closer and closer approximations to the desired goal (long-term retention over days, weeks, and months) intrinsically reinforced through successfully recalling target information (Camp, Bird, & Cherry, 2000).

We chose SR, in conjunction with the use of external aids, as an intervention for the current pilot study for several reasons. First, we have had success using SR to enable persons with mild to severe memory deficits secondary to a wide range of etiologies, including Alzheimer's disease and other dementing conditions, to learn and retain new information over long time intervals (days, weeks, and months), while enhancing their capacity to function more independently (see Camp et al., 2000, for review). Second, we have seen SR used successfully in case studies of older adults with Parkinson's disease with dementia (Hayden & Camp, 1995). Cognitive deficits seen in persons who are HIV+ strongly resemble the neuropsychological deficits associated with Parkinson's disease (PD), specifically, slowness of thought and motor activity (see Bartok et al., 1997; Martin et al., 1993). Third, we have seen SR used effectively at our own facility, Menorah Park, with younger adults with executive dysfunction due to Traumatic Brain Injury (TBI).

Further support for selecting SR as the intervention comes from evidence that successful recall following SR training contrasts sharply with most other attempts (e.g., cueing hierarchies) by persons with memory deficits to remember recent information (Bourgeois et al., 2003). In addition, learning through SR seems to take place with little or no expenditure of cognitive effort on the part of the learner (Camp et al., 2000). SR can be embedded within the context of a social visit or standard therapy sessions, e.g., speech-language therapy (Brush & Camp, 1998a, 1998b), thus creating a positive experience while at the same time providing success in learning and remembering new information. For all these reasons, we hypothesized that SR would be an effective intervention for cognitive deficits in persons aged 50 and over with HIV.

In preliminary work for the present study, Lee and Camp (2001) showed that SR was an effective cognitive intervention with two older adults with HIV who demonstrated memory impairments, one with mild impairment and the other with moderate to severe impairment. Although both persons were initially unable to recall, after an hour delay, newly presented target information (e.g., the name of a person and a 3-step verbal-motor response), following SR training, both were able to recall the information across multiple days. With further testing and simplification of the protocol, we expect that SR could be embedded within a clinic visit as part of education sessions conducted by case managers, social workers, nurses or other health professionals to teach persons with HIV to take their medications correctly and remember their clinic appointments. We have recent preliminary data supporting the effectiveness of SR delivered over the telephone (Joltin, Camp, & McMahon, 2003), a technique that, with further refinement, would increase the feasibility of delivering this intervention within busy clinic settings.

METHOD

Participants

The study was approved for protection of human subjects by the Institutional Review Board of Menorah Park Center for Senior Living. Study participants included 17 HIV positive persons aged 50 or over who were referred by clinicians and service providers, including doctors and nurses at HIV/AIDS clinics, visiting nurses providing HIV/AIDS home visits, and HIV/AIDS case managers at social service agencies. Criteria for referral were: (1) age 50 and over; (2) diagnosis of HIV or AIDS; (3) medically stable; (4) able to speak, read, and write English; and (5) able to physically manipulate experimental materials. Although clinicians were told that neurocognitive testing would determine if the participant met criteria for cognitive deficits, clinicians tended to refer participants whom they thought were having at least some memory problems. Clinicians gave potential participants initial information about the study and then obtained permission for the project manager to call them and explain the study in detail. Of the 24 persons initially referred for the study, 3 decided not to participate for unknown reasons, 2 were not able to schedule study visits around work commitments, one became too ill, and one died, leaving 17 participants who began the study. At the first home visit, a study staff member reviewed the consent form and obtained the participant's signed consent. Fifteen participants completed all three required screening sessions. One participant was excluded because of active alcohol abuse and the other because he cancelled two consecutive appointments. Of the 15 who completed screening, 13 met the criterion for executive function deficits. Three of the latter did not continue the study: two could not be contacted for the treatment phase and one became too ill. The final sample receiving the intervention, therefore, included 10 participants.

The mean age of the 10 participants was 53 years (range 50-60 years). There were 7 men and 3 women, including 5 Whites and 5 African Americans; one was Hispanic; years of education ranged from 11 to 19 years. Five participants lived alone; three were in an HIV/AIDS adult group home; one lived with a partner; and one lived with his teenage son. All participants were unemployed. Except for one white, male subject living in a middle-class suburb, all could be characterized as urban poor.

Participants had been diagnosed with HIV/AIDS from one year to over 10 years. Seven of the 10 participants had AIDS. Three had CD4 cells/cu mm of less than 200; 2 were in the CD4 range of 201-350; and 5 had CD4 counts over 350. All participants were taking highly active antiretroviral therapy (HAART), except one participant who had been diagnosed within the last year. Participants had multiple co-morbidities, similar to samples of non-HIV infected persons aged 65 or over, including hypertension, strokes, and heart disease. Four had been treated for drug abuse in the past, three had been treated for alcohol abuse and four were currently being treated for depression. Thus, this sample represented the heterogeneity of the "real world" of people aged 50 and over living with HIV.

Design

The design included administration of an initial battery of neuropsychological tests conducted in the participant's home, by a PhD in clinical psychology with special training in assessment of older persons, who was assisted by one of two research associates who were trained in administering the tests. All sessions were conducted by two of these three staff persons, with the majority of the sessions led by the PhD; the research associate collected demographics and the medical history and either administered, set up or timed the tests. Participants were paid $10 per session. Those participants who met the criterion for executive function deficits were referred to the intervention phase of the study.

In the intervention phase, participants selected two functional goals (e.g., remembering to take medications and remembering clinic appointments) and self-reported their baseline difficulty with these functions. Then, appropriate cue/response sets (e.g., "What do you do when you take your medications?" "I check them off the checklist.") were selected by participants with guidance from the SR therapists. An external aid that would assist each participant (e.g., checklist, timer) with each functional goal also was selected collaboratively.

Two research staff members, a speech therapist and a research associate, both with training in administering SR, conducted the intervention in 1/2 hour training sessions, typically twice a week over 4 weeks (or across 8 treatment sessions). All sessions were conducted in the participant's home so as to assure that the intervention was appropriate and acceptable within the setting where the participant would be using the intervention. For most sessions, both staff members were present, but depending on the safety of the participant's neighborhood and the ease with which the participant learned the intervention, the research associate would independently conduct the training. Participants were paid $5 for each training session. Two months after the last training session, with no intervening contact with participants, the SR therapists conducted the post-treatment assessment, including participants' self-report of the training's effectiveness, test of recall of the correct SR responses and evidence of use of the external aids. Participants were paid $20 for the post-treatment assessment.

Screening Measures and Results

The screening was conducted over three sessions, all in the participant's home, with each session designed to last approximately one hour to avoid excessively fatiguing the participant. Screening instruments were selected based on:

(1) recommendation by the National Institute of Mental Health (NIMH) Workshop on neuropsychological assessment of AIDS-related cognitive changes (Butters et al., 1990) and/or (2) identification by Bryan and Luszcz (2000) as suitable for detecting age differences in executive function. Table 1 lists all of the measures used in the study.

Neuropsychological Deficits

The operational criterion for executive function deficits used in this study was a score at least one standard deviation below the mean for normative samples of older persons on at least one of the following three tests (see Table 2 for descriptive statistics on all screening measures):

(1) *The California Verbal Learning Test-Semantic Clustering Ratio* (CVLT) (Delis, Kramer, Kaplan, & Ober, 1987) is a test of memory and learning efficiency based on the degree to which the participant uses a "mental filing system" for reorganizing the target words (e.g., apricots) into categorical groups (e.g., fruit), which typically results in the most efficient learning strategy. With raw scores of 0 and above indicating more efficient learning, raw scores in this sample ranged from 0.3 to 2.3, which converted to standard scores, based on tabled norms for age and gender, that ranged from -2 to 0 (normal), with 7 participants scoring in the study deficit range.

(2) *The Modified Wisconsin Card Sorting Test-Number of Perseverative Errors* (MCST) (Hart, Kwentus, Wade, & Taylor, 1988 modification) assesses problem solving ability and cognitive flexibility (Bryan & Luszcz, 2000). A perseverative error is scored when the participant persists with an incorrect response after feedback. In this sample, raw scores ranged widely from 0 (no perseverative errors) to 71 errors, which converted to standard scores, based on age and education, that ranged from within normal limits to the highly severe deficit range (-14). Seven participants scored in the study deficit range.

(3) A test of verbal fluency, the *FAS-Test* (Spreen & Strauss, 1998), which is one of the most widely used tests of executive function, measures the speed and ease of verbal production and assesses the readiness with which participants can initiate behavior in response to a novel request (Bryan & Luszcz, 2000). Participants were asked to generate as many words as possible beginning with the letters F, A, and S. Raw scores on total number of correct words ranged from 14 to 55, which converted to standard scores based on age that ranged from -2.25 to within normal limits, with 5 subjects scoring in the study deficit range.

Two participants scored in the study deficit range on all three of the above tests; four had deficits on two tests; and three participants had deficits on only one test (two on the CVLT and 1 on the MCST). These three tests were selected as the criterion measures because norms for persons aged 50 and over were available and they were sensitive to deficits in this sample.

TABLE 1. Neuropsychological Instruments

Session 1

Depression	Hamilton Depression Inventory (HamD) (Hamilton, 1960; Reynolds & Kobak, 1995)
Anxiety	State-Trait Anxiety Inventory (STAI) (Spielberger, Gorsuch, Lushene, Vagg & Jacobs, 1983)
Dementia	HIV Dementia Scale (HDS) (Power, Selnes, Grim, & McArthur, 1995)
Memory/Learning	California Verbal Learning Test (CVLT) (Delis, Kramer, Kaplan, & Ober, 1987)
Attention	Wechsler Memory Scale – 3rd Edition Spatial Span (WMS-III) (Wechsler, 1997)

Session 2

Abstraction	Modified Wisconsin Card Sorting Test (MCST) (Hart, Kwentus, Wade, & Taylor, 1988)
Flexibility	Uses for Objects (Bryan & Luszcz, 2000; Getzels & Jackson, 1962)
Dementia	The Mini-Mental Status Examination (MMSE) (Folstein, Folstein, & McHugh, 1975)
Premorbid Intelligence	Wechsler Adult Intelligence Scale – III -Vocabulary (WAIS – III) (Wechsler, 1997)

Session 3

Planning	Tower of London Test (Shallice, 1982)
Monitoring	Self-Ordered Pointing Task (SOPT) (Petrides & Milner, 1982)
Concentration	Stroop Color and Word Test (SCWT) (Daigneault, Braun, & Whitaker, 1992)
Language, Novelty	Verbal Fluency Test (FAS) (Spreen & Strauss, 1998)
Language, Novelty	Excluded Letter Fluency (ELF) (Bryan, Luszcz, & Crawford, 1997)

We tested general mental status of participants with: (1) *HIV Dementia Scale* (HDS) (Power, Selnes, Grim, & McArthur, 1995), which measures cognitive functioning in areas in which patients with mild HIV dementia have significant deficits, including attention, psychomotor speed, memory-recall and visual-spatial construction. Scores on the HDS may range from 0 to 16, with a score of ≤ 10 indicating dementia. In this sample, scores ranged from 3.5 to 15, with 4 participants scoring in the HIV dementia range. (2) *The Mini-Mental Status Examination* (MMSE) (Folstein, Folstein, & McHugh, 1975), which is a standard measure of cognitive function that, in comparison to the HDS, has better norms for older populations and persons with low education and is less sensitive to psychomotor slowing since performance is not timed. Scores on the MMSE may range from 0 to 30, with scores of ≤ 23 indicating dementia. In this sample, MMSE scores ranged from 18 to 30 with 2 participants scoring in the dementia range.

TABLE 2. Descriptive Statistics on Neuropsychological Tests (Raw Scores) and Number of Participants Meeting Deficit Criterion and Clinical Cutoff Scores

Screening Test	Mean	SD	Min / Max	Number with Deficit	N
CVLT	1.4	0.7	0.3 / 2.3	7	9[a]
MCST	26.9	27.9	0.0 / 71.0	7	10
FAS	35.4	11.5	14.0 / 55.0	5	10
HDS	10.5	3.7	3.5 / 15.0	4	10
MMSE	25.3	3.5	18.0 / 30.0	2	10
HamD	19.2	11.5	7.5 / 35.5	4	10
StAnx	39.4	12.2	21.0 / 57.0	5	10
TrAnx	34.5	10.9	20.0 / 54.0	4	10

Note. CVLT = California Verbal Learning Test (Semantic Cluster Ratio); MCST = Modified Wisconsin Card Sort Test (Number of Perseverative Errors); FAS = Verbal Fluency Test (Total Number Correct); HDS = HIV Dementia Scale; MMSE = Mini-Mental Status Exam; HamD = Hamilton Depression Inventory; StAnx = State-Trait Anxiety Inventory (State Anxiety); TrAnx = State-Trait Anxiety Inventory (Trait Anxiety).
[a]One participant did not complete the CVLT

Clearly, in this sample, the MMSE and the HDS were not as sensitive to early cognitive deficits as the CVLT, the MCST, or the FAS, especially for those deficits related to executive function.

The *Hamilton Depression Inventory* (HamD) (Hamilton, 1960; Reynolds & Kobak, 1995) was used to measure depression, a common effect of HIV, opportunistic infections and some HIV medications, and an often-reported predictor of failure to take medications (Perry & Karasic, 2002). In this sample, the range of scores was 7.5 to 35.5, with 4 participants scoring at 19 or above, the cutoff for at least mild depressive symptomatology. The *State-Trait Anxiety Inventory* (STAI) (Spielberger, Gorsuch, Lushene, Vagg, & Jacobs, 1983) was used to measure state anxiety (transitory) and trait anxiety (a relatively stable personality feature) since anxiety may impair memory and learning. Five participants scored with at least mild/moderate trait anxiety and four scored with at least mild/moderate trait anxiety. Depression and anxiety, therefore, were factors that could potentially impair participants' memory and learning abilities.

The only significant zero-order correlations among the above neuropsychological tests were the following (see Table 3): both the HIV Dementia Scale (HDS) and the MMSE were correlated with more perseverative errors on the MCST ($r = -.66$ and $-.64$, respectively); the HDS and MMSE were highly correlated (.70); higher trait and state anxiety were correlated with lower scores on the HDS (more dementia), and the measures of anxiety and depression were highly inter-correlated. With a larger sample, other correlations, such as between the CVLT and HDS (.53) and the FAS and HDS (.43), might have reached significance. The few significant inter-correlations in this sample might be interpreted as confirming that these measures were tapping relatively discrete cognitive functions.

Treatment Goals, Process and Outcome Measures

At the first treatment visit, the two SR therapists identified participants' individual goals for the intervention by asking participants what kinds of things they would like to work on during "memory training." Nine out of 10 participants self-selected two goals; one participant selected only one goal. The goals and number of participants selecting them were: remember appointments (7), remember medications (5), remember today's date (2), remember to eat (1), remember to pay bills (1), remember phone numbers (1), remember to cross off words for a word search (1), and find a positive article in the newspaper each morning (1). (This last goal was used for a participant who complained of feeling depressed.) Each participant used one external aid per goal, except for one participant who used two aids for the second goal. Five participants used pill organizers to help remember medications; seven used calendars to help keep appointments; four used timers that allow multiple settings for one day; three used checklists; two used newspapers (one participant searched for a positive article and another used it to identify the date); one used a cue card; one used a rolodex; and one used an expandable file folder to help keep track of bills and receipts.

Each participant was trained on one goal at a time, with training for each goal typically lasting four complete sessions. During training sessions, participants tried to recall responses and procedures over progressively expanding

TABLE 3. Pearson Correlations Among Neuropsychological Tests Raw Scores

	CVLT	MCST	FAS	HDS	MMSE	HamD	TrAnx	StAnx
CVLT								
MCST	−.21							
FAS	.09	−.41						
HDS	.53	−.66*	.43					
MMSE	−.06	−.64*	.14	.70*				
HamD	.04	−.24	.37	.51	.22			
TrAnx	.37	−.33	.42	.71*	.28	.93**		
StAnx	.08	−.53	.54	−.67*	.37	.87**	.85**	

*p < 0.05 level (2-tailed).
**p < 0.01 level (2-tailed).

time intervals, beginning with 30 sec, then 1 min, 2 min, 4 min, 8 min, and 16 min. Participants also were trained when and how to appropriately use the external aids (e.g., setting the timer). If participants erred, they were provided the correct response, and asked to immediately recall it. The subsequent trial then involved re-recalling the response over a time period equal to that of the last successfully recalled trial (e.g., if the participant erred at 4 min, the next trial recall was at 2 min). After the initial training session, each subsequent session began with the therapist querying the participant about the target response (e.g., "What do you do when the timer goes off?" "Take my medications and turn off the timer"). If participants were unable to recall the correct response, training would resume, beginning with the delay equal to that of the last successful recall obtained in the previous session. Training for each goal ended when initial mastery was achieved; initial mastery was defined as a participant giving the correct response at the start of three consecutive training sessions spaced 2-5 days apart.

"Retention" of mastery was measured two months post-treatment, with no intervening contact or "booster" training with participants. Retention was indicated by the following outcome measures: (1) the participant giving the correct response to the cue at the two-month post-treatment session; (2) the therapist identifying an objective indication of current use of the procedure (e.g., medications were checked off the list, the timer was in place, the pill counter was visible and up-to-date, etc.); (3) the participant reporting that the treatment had a positive effect on his/her ability to meet the designated goal (e.g., remember to take medications).

A case example illustrates the SR training. Mr. R was a 52-year-old, extremely thin, white male, who had completed high school and worked most of his life as a waiter and bartender. He was diagnosed with AIDS approximately four years prior to the first study visit. His CD4 count was 80 cells/cu. mm. and his viral load (HIV RNA, standard PCR) was 2630 copies/ml.[3] He was on HAART and an anti-depressant. Mr. R denied past or current drug or alcohol abuse, but reported currently drinking 2-3 beers a day. He reported taking medications for depression for about two months in the prior year. He lived with a supportive male partner in a subsidized housing apartment. His MMSE was 18/30; HDS was 6/16, and he scored in the severe deficit range on the WCST, with 71 perseverative errors (standard score = −14); his CVLT Semantic Ratio score was within normal limits (although he scored in the deficit range on other CVLT measures focused on memory); and his FAS total number of words correct was 24 (standard score = −1.42). He did not score as either depressed or anxious.

Mr. R's first goal was to remember to eat. The detailed treatment goal was that Mr. R would use a timer, provided and set by the research staff (his partner was trained to reset it, if needed), that would buzz every day at 8AM, 1PM, and 5PM. He was trained on the following cue/response: "What do you do when the buzzer goes off?" "Turn off the buzzer and prepare to eat." The procedure was that he would turn off the timer, get out a placemat, plate and silverware, which were visual cues to eat. At the first training session, he demonstrated the correct response 5/7 trials, remembering it for a maximum of 8 minutes. At the next three training sessions, spaced between 2-5 days later, he remembered the correct response on the initial trial at each of the three sessions, which indicated that he had achieved initial mastery. At the two-month follow-up, he did not provide the correct verbal response to the prompt question, but the timer was set correctly and the placemat was visible, although Mr. R had moved to a new apartment in the interim. He and his partner reported that the treatment was effective and he was eating more frequently.

Mr. R's second goal was to remember to take his medications. He reported "a little difficulty" remembering medications, but his partner reported that he was having a great deal of difficulty, confirmed by the number of pills in a jar where Mr. R had "hidden" his missed doses. He did not use a pill organizer; rather, he said that he remembered to take his medications "in his head." The treatment goal was that Mr. R would use a checklist to check off his medications when he had taken them. The cue/response was, "What do you do after you have taken your meds? " "Check them off the list." At the first training session, he demonstrated the correct response 4/10 trials, remembering it for a maximum of 30 sec. At the session #2, he remembered the cue/response 6/8 trials, remembering it for a maximum of 8 min. At the next two sessions, he demonstrated initial mastery. At the two-month follow-up, he provided the correct verbal response, demonstrated appropriate use of the checklist (and previously used checklists were observed by the research assistant to be appropriately checked off), and both he and his partner reported that his medication adherence had improved.

RESULTS

As shown in Table 4, for goal #1, the number of participants achieving initial mastery of the correct response and procedure was 9/10. The one participant who did not achieve mastery of the single goal he chose had requested a change in response and procedure twice. The therapists offered suggestions, but the participant chose not to follow through with them. Therefore, we terminated further training for this participant, but included him in the post-treatment evaluation. All 9 participants who achieved initial mastery on goal #1 did so within 4 training sessions. For goal #1, at the post-treatment evaluation, 6/10 participants gave the correct response, thus demonstrating that they had retained mastery over two months. All 10 participants, including the one who did not achieve initial mastery, self-reported that the treatment for goal #1 was effective. For all 10 participants, therapists noted objective signs (e.g., timer in place and set, medications checked off the list, etc.) that the participant was using the external aid for goal #1. For goal #2, all 9 participants who had selected a second goal achieved initial mastery. Eight participants achieved initial mastery in 4 training sessions and one did so in 5 sessions. For goal #2, at the post-treatment evaluation, 8/9 participants gave the correct response, thus demonstrating two-month retention of mastery. All 9 participants subjectively reported that the treatment for goal #2 was effective and therapists noted objective signs that all 9 participants were using the external aid.

DISCUSSION

Results of this pilot study demonstrated the potential of a cognitive intervention to compensate for cognitive deficits among persons aged 50 and over with HIV/AIDS. Of the 10 persons who identified at least one goal (e.g., remembering appointments), 9 initially mastered the correct response and procedure; 6 retained the correct response and procedure at the two-month posttreatment evaluation, demonstrating retention of mastery; and all 10 self-reported that the intervention had helped them achieve their goal. Among the 9 persons who identified a second goal, all 9 initially mastered the correct response and procedure; 8 retained them at the post-treatment evaluation, demonstrating retention of mastery; and all 9 reported that the intervention was effective. These results were achieved among persons with a broad range of cognitive deficits.

The results from this pilot study have several important implications regarding cognitive deficits in HIV+ older adults. The first is that, though the sample was small, a surprisingly large percentage of these persons presented with cognitive deficits that can affect the ability to follow complex care regimens. Of the 15 participants who completed the full battery for cognitive screening, 13 met the operational criteria for executive function deficits. Of the 10 who went on to the intervention phase of the study, 7 self-identified problems with keeping track of appointments and 5 self-identified problems with remembering to take their medications. These numbers may represent underreporting of these problems, since lack of insight and failure to accurately monitor performance are typical in persons with executive dysfunction.

TABLE 4. Ratio of Participants (number/sample) Achieving Initial Mastery and 2 Month Retention

	Achieved Initial Mastery	Two Month Follow-Up		
		Gave Correct Verbal Response	Reported Effectiveness	Procedure in Use
Goal #1	9/10	6/10	10/10	10/10
Goal #2	9/9	8/9	9/9	9/9

Given that most persons in our sample did not have caregivers who lived with them, we could corroborate participants' self-reports of deficits and self-reports of treatment effectiveness with only one caregiver, the partner of Mr. R in the case example. That caregiver reported that, pre-treatment, the participant was having significantly greater difficulties with remembering medications than the participant himself reported, but that the treatment had indeed improved his medication adherence. Although the sample was small, not randomly selected, nor compared to a control group, this pattern of results suggests that older HIV+ adults have significant difficulties regarding their ability to monitor and maintain health-promoting behaviors. They are particularly challenged in the areas of adherence to medication regimens and keeping clinic appointments. This may be especially true of persons without the social support provided by a live-in companion/caregiver.

The second implication is that providing external aids (pill organizers, calendars) appears insufficient to enable HIV+ older adults to overcome executive dysfunction. Although we did not study a group that was using external aids without SR, all five participants who reported difficulty with taking medications already had pill organizers, but they were unable to use them effectively. With adherence rates of 95% to HAART (highly active anti-retroviral treatment) recommended to achieve optimized virologic outcomes (Paterson et al., 2000), if compliance is not maintained, there is increased risk of drug resistance and drug failure (Nieuwkerk et al., 2001). The likelihood of transmission of drug-resistant strains of HIV is increased for persons with HIV and executive function deficits, including difficulties with planning/anticipating, judgment and self-monitoring (Bryan & Luszcz, 2000; Ferrer-Caja, Crawford, & Bryan, 2002), since these deficits not only interfere with adherence but with consistent HIV/AIDS prevention behaviors. Thus, non-pharmacological interventions that can allow external aids to be used most effectively to improve adherence are critically important from a public health perspective.

The third implication is that the use of SR, in conjunction with external aids, shows promise for enabling HIV+ older adults to compensate for executive function deficits and to improve adherence to care regimens. Positive SR treatment effects were demonstrated across a wide range of cognitive status levels, including individuals with AIDS and test scores indicative of the presence of dementia. In addition, SR was effective in HIV+ older adults who presented with scores indicative of clinical depression, and it was even used to develop an intervention to help combat depression. SR goals were also relatively well preserved over the two-month follow-up time, in spite of the absence of "booster sessions" or maintenance training that would be part of standard rehabilitation practices.

Clinical implications, especially for case managers and social workers, include the need to recognize early signs of HIV-associated cognitive deficits, especially symptoms of executive dysfunction in the absence of diagnosed dementia. This is important because such deficits can significantly impair clients' ability to keep appointments, adhere to medication regimens, follow-up on service recommendations and apply for benefits. When the case manager suspects cognitive dysfunction, referrals for neuropsychological testing should be made so that cognitive deficits, as well as preserved abilities, can be identified and appropriate treatments, including SR, can be instituted. We would recommend that social workers in the field of HIV/AIDS, who undoubtedly will be seeing older clients more frequently in the future, consult with social workers, nurses and physicians who specialize in geriatrics and make linkages with agencies that provide services for older persons. For example, the Alzheimer's Association, nationally and locally, could be a good source for dementia-specific educational material and services. Also, agencies providing services for those with traumatic brain injury and other patient groups with executive dysfunction could be good contacts. Knowledge shared among those in the fields of HIV/AIDS, aging, substance abuse, and mental health would greatly benefit older persons with HIV/AIDS. This sharing would help break down many cross-field stereotypes about older persons, those with dementia, and people with HIV/AIDS, histories of substance abuse, and/or mental illness. Such sharing could foster development of new service programs, as well as much needed cross-disciplinary research.

This study represents a pilot project and an initial attempt to determine the feasibility of this type of intervention. Future studies will focus on developing a larger sample size, adding appropriate control groups, and comparing effects produced by SR versus other cognitive interventions, as well as external aids, such as pill organizers, alone. Comparisons of effects across age groups, including younger persons with HIV/AIDS, would also strengthen the generalizability of the results. We would add additional objective baseline and outcome measures (e.g., does viral load significantly decrease?) and extend the follow-up period from 2 months to at least 9 months to assure a longer retention effect. We would recommend both baseline and follow-up neuropsychological testing. The length of each testing session should be limited to approximately one hour and be conducted at the clinic site to reduce staff cost and improve consistency of testing conditions. The assessment would include the CVLT (Delis et al., 1987) and the MCST (Hart et al., 1988), our most sensitive measures; other tests that we would recommend for consideration would be the Trail Making Test (Spreen & Strauss, 1998) and the Clock Drawing Test (Spreen & Strauss, 1998).

Further refinement of the SR training protocol would focus on simplifying it to make it more feasible for harried case managers, social workers, and other staff to conduct within the demanding environments of HIV/AIDS care. Since the series of home visits for SR delivery described in this study is not likely to be feasible in most care environments, we are currently testing the delivery of the protocol entirely within the clinic setting. Also, since preliminary data supports the effectiveness of SR training delivered over the telephone (Joltin et al., 2003), we will compare in-person delivery of the SR intervention with SR delivery over the telephone. In this future study, subjects will be randomly assigned to either treatment group or to a wait-list control group that receives standard clinic adherence education. These results will further test the effectiveness and feasibility of this cognitive intervention.

Despite the limitations of this pilot study, the findings suggest that a cognitive intervention based in SR techniques deserves to be further studied for its potential as an adjunct to pharmacological intervention in HIV+ older adults. With further refinement and testing, health care providers, including case managers, social workers, nurses and even non-professionals, such as home health aides and family caregivers, could be trained to deliver SR treatments to clients so as to improve their adherence to HIV/AIDS care regimens.

REFERENCES

Bartok, J. A., Martin, E. M., Pitrak, D. L., Novak, R. M., Pursell, K. J., Mullane, K. M. et al. (1997). Working memory deficits in HIV-seropositive drug users. *Journal of the International Neuropsychological Society, 3*, 451-456.

Bourgeois, M. S., Camp, C. J., Rose, M., White, B., Malone, M., Carr, J. et al. (2003). A comparison of training strategies to enhance use of external aids by persons with dementia. *Journal of Communication Disorders.*

Brush, J. A., & Camp, C. J. (1998a). Using spaced-retrieval as an intervention during speech-language therapy. *Clinical Gerontologist, 19,* 51-64.

Brush, J. A., & Camp, C. J. (1998b). Using spaced retrieval to treat dysphagia in a long-term care resident with dementia. *Clinical Gerontologist, 19 (2),* 96-99.

Bryan, J., & Luszcz, M. A. (2000). Measurement of executive function: Considerations for detecting adult age differences. *Journal of Clinical and Experimental Neuropsychology, 22(1),* 40-55.

Bryan, J., Luszcz, M. A., & Crawford, J. R. (1997). Verbal knowledge and speed of information processing as mediators of age differences in verbal fluency performance among older adults. *Psychology and Aging, 12,* 473-478.

Butters, N., Grant, I., Haxby, J., Judd, L. L., Martin, A., McClelland, J., Pequegnat, W., Schacter, D., & Stover, E. (1990). Assessment of AIDS-related cognitive changes: Recommendations of the NIMH workshop on neuropsychological assessment approaches. *Journal of Clinical and Experimental Neuropsychology, 12,* 963-978.

Camp, C. J., Bird, M. J., & Cherry, K. E. (2000). Retrieval strategies as a rehabilitation aid for cognitive loss in pathological aging. In R. D. Hill, L. Bäckman, & A. S. Neely (Eds.), *Cognitive rehabilitation in old age,* 224-248. New York: Oxford University Press.

Castellon, S. A., Hinkin, C. H., & Myers, H. F. (2000). Neuropsychiatric disturbance is associated with executive dysfunction in HIV-1 infection. *Journal of the International Neuropsychological Society, 6,* 336-347.

CDC, Center for Disease Control, 2003. Retrieved from http://www.cdc.gov/hiv/stats/hasrsupp91/table2.htm

Daigneault, S., Braun, M. J., & Whitaker, H. A. (1992). Early effects of normal aging on perseverative and non-perseverative prefrontal measures. *Developmental Neuropsychology, 8,* 99-114.

Delis, D. C., Kramer, J. H., Kaplan, E., & Ober, B. A. (1987). *CVLT, California Verbal Learning Test Manual* (Version 1). San Antonio: The Psychological Corporation, Harcourt Brace.

Emlet, C. A., & Farkas, K. J. (2001). A descriptive analysis of older adults with HIV/AIDS in California. *Health & Social Work, 26,* 226-234.

Ferrer-Caja, E., Crawford, J. R., & Bryan, J. (2002). A structural modeling examination of the executive decline hypothesis of cognitive aging through reanalysis of Crawford et al.'s (2000) data. *Aging, Neuropsychology, and Cognition, 9,* 231-249.

Folstein, M. F., Folstein, S. E., & McHugh, P. R. (1975). "Mini-mental state": A practical method for grading the cognitive state of patients for the clinician. *Journal of Psychiatric Research, 12,* 189-198.

Getzels, J. W., & Jackson, P. W. (1962). *Creativity and intelligence.* New York: Wiley.

Goldenberg, D., & Boyle, B. (2000). Psychiatry and HIV: Part 2. *AIDS Reader, 10,* 201-204.

Goodkin, K., Wilkie, F. L., Hinkin, C. H., Symes, S., Baldewicz, T. T., Asthana, D. et al. (2001). Aging and neuro-AIDS conditions and the changing spectrum of HIV-1-associated morbidity and mortality. *Journal of Clinical Epidemiology, 54,* S35-S43.

Hamilton, M. (1960). A rating scale for depression. *Journal of Neurology, Neurosurgery, and Psychiatry, 23,* 56-62.

Hart, R. P., Kwentus, J. A., Wade, J. B., & Taylor, J. R. (1988). Modified Wisconsin Sorting Test in elderly normal, depressed and demented patients. *The Clinical Neuropsychologist, 2,* 49-56.

Hayden, C. M., & Camp, C. J. (1995). Spaced-retrieval: A memory intervention for dementia in Parkinson's disease. *Clinical Gerontologist, 16(2),* 80-82.

Heckman, T. G., Kochman, A., Sikkema, K. J., Kalichman, S. C., Masten, J., & Goodkin, K. (2000). Late middle-aged and older men living with HIV/AIDS: Race differences in coping, social support, and psychological distress. *Journal of the National Medical Association, 92,* 436-444.

Joltin, A., Camp, C. J., & McMahon, C. M. (2003). Spaced-retrieval over the telephone: An intervention for persons with dementia. *Clinical Psychologist, 7(1),* 50-55.

Koutsilieri, E., ter Meulen, V., & Riederer, P. (2001). Neurotransmission in HIV associated dementia: A short review. *Journal of Neural Transmission, 108,* 767-775.

Lee, M., & Camp, C. J. (2001). Spaced-retrieval: A memory intervention for HIV+ older adults. *Clinical Gerontologist, 22(3/4),* 131-135.

Libon, D. J., Glosser, G., Malamut, B. L., Kaplan, E., Goldberg, E., Swenson, R., & Sands, L. P. (1994). Age, executive functions, and visuospatial functioning in healthy older adults. *Neuropsychology, 8(1),* 38-43.

Linsk, N. L. (2000). HIV among older adults: Age-specific issues in prevention and treatment. *AIDS Reader, 10,* 430-444.

Mack, K. A., & Bland, S. D. (1999). HIV testing behaviors and attitudes regarding HIV/AIDS of adults aged 50-64. *The Gerontologist, 39,* 687-694.

Martin, A., Heyes, M. P., Salazar, A. M., Law, W. A., & Williams, J. (1993). Impaired motor-skill learning, slowed reaction time, and elevated cerebrospinal fluid quinolinic acid in a group of HIV-infected individuals. *Neuropsychology, 7,* 149-157.

Martin, E. M., Pitrak, D. L., Robertson, L. C., Novak, R. M., Mullane, K. M., & Pursell, K. J. (1995). Global-local analysis in HIV-1 infection. *Neuropsychology, 9,* 102-109.

Martin, E. M., Pitrak, D. L., Pursell, K. J., Mullan, K. M., & Novak, R. M. (1995). Delayed recognition memory span in HIV-1 infection. *Journal of the International Neuropsychological Society, 1,* 575-580.

Martin, E. M., Pitrak, D. L., Rains, N., Grbesic, S., Pursell, K., Nunnally, G., & Bechara, A. (2003). Delayed nonmatch-to-sample performance in HIV-seropositive and HIV-seronegative polydrug abusers. *Neuropsychology, 17,* 283-288.

Nieuwkerk, P. T., Sprangers, M. A., Burger, D. M., Hoetelmans, R. M., Hugen, P. W., Danner, S. A. et al. (2001). Limited patient adherence to highly active antiretroviral therapy for HIV-1 infection in an observational cohort study. *Archives of Internal Medicine, 161* (16), 1962-1968.

Ory, M. G., & Mack, K. A. (1998). Middle-aged and older people with AIDS. *Research on Aging, 20,* 653-664.

Paterson, D. L., Swindells, S., Mohr, J. et al. (2000). Adherence to protease inhibitor therapy and outcomes in patients with HIV infection. *Annals of Internal Medicine, 133,* 21-30.

Perry, S., & Karasic, D. (2002). Depression, adherence to HAART, and survival. *Focus, A Guide to AIDS Research and Counseling, AIDS Health Project, 17 (9),* 5-6.

Petrides, M., & Milner, B. (1982). Deficits on subject-ordered tasks after frontal and temporal-lobe lesions in man. *Neurospychologia, 20,* 249-262.

Power, C., Selnes, O., Grim, J., & McArthur, J. (1995). HIV Dementia Scale: A rapid screening test. *Journal of Acquired Immune Deficiency Syndromes and Human Retrovirology, 8(3),* 273-278.

Reynolds, W. M. & Kobak, K. A. (1995). *HDI: Hamilton depression inventory, a self-report version of the Hamilton Depression Rating Scale, Professional Manual.* Odessa, FL: Psychological Assessment Resources.

Salthouse, T. A., Fristoe, N., & Rhee, S. H. (1996). How localized are age-related effects on neuropsychological measures. *Neuropsychology, 10(2),* 272-285.

Shallice, T. (1982). Specific impairments of planning. *Philosophical Transactions of the Royal Society of London, 298B,* 199-209.

Spielberger, C. D., Gorsuch, R. L., Lushene, R., Vagg, P. R., & Jacobs, G. A. (1983). *State-Trait Anxiety Inventory for Adults.* Redwood City, CA: Mind Garden.

Spreen, O. & Strauss, E. (1998). *A compendium of neuropsychological tests.* 447-459. New York: Oxford University Press.

Taylor, M. J., Alhassoon, O. M., Schweinsburg, B. S., Videen, J. S., Grant, I., & The HNRC Group. (2000). MR spectroscopy in HIV and stimulant dependence. *Journal of the International Neuropsychological Society, 6,* 83-85.

Wechsler, D. (1997). WMS-III Administration and Scoring Manual. San Antonio: Harcourt Brace & Co.

White, F. L., Heaton, R. K., Monsch, A. U., and the HIV Neurobehavioral Research Group (1995). Neuropsychological studies of asymptomatic human immunodeficiency virus-type-1 infected individuals. *Journal of the International Neuropsychological Society, 1,* 304-315.

Winocur, G., Moscovitch, M., & Stuss, D. T. (1996). Explicit and implicit memory in the elderly: Evidence for double dissociation involving medial temporal and frontal lobe functions. *Neuropsychology, 10(1),* 57-65.

Six Champions Speak
About Being Over 50
and Living with HIV

Cynthia Cannon Poindexter, PhD, MSW

SUMMARY. One-time telephone interviews were conducted with six middle-aged and older HIV-positive advocates who spoke about their views on the intersection of AIDS and aging. Despite their diversity, the participants spoke similarly about support, stigma, activism, health maintenance, the difficulty of separating the effects of HIV from the effects of aging, and a renewed gratitude about life and love. *[Article copies available for a fee from The Haworth Document Delivery Service: 1-800-HAWORTH. E-mail address: <docdelivery@haworthpress.com> Website: <http://www.HaworthPress.com> © 2004 by The Haworth Press, Inc. All rights reserved.]*

KEYWORDS. HIV, AIDS, aging

The HIV field has a tradition of inclusion of those who are affected and infected, and social work is predicated on empowerment and self-determination. Therefore it seemed necessary to incorporate in this volume some voices of middle-aged and older persons who are living with HIV. To that end, between

Cynthia Cannon Poindexter, PhD, MSW, is Associate Professor at Fordham University Graduate School of Social Service.

[Haworth co-indexing entry note]: "Six Champions Speak About Being Over 50 and Living with HIV." Poindexter, Cynthia Cannon. Co-published simultaneously in *Journal of HIV/AIDS & Social Services* (The Haworth Press) Vol. 3, No. 1, 2004, pp. 99-117; and: *Midlife and Older Adults and HIV: Implications for Social Service Research, Practice, and Policy* (ed: Cynthia Cannon Poindexter, and Sharon M. Keigher) The Haworth Press, Inc., 2004, pp. 99-117. Single or multiple copies of this article are available for a fee from The Haworth Document Delivery Service [1-800-HAWORTH, 9:00 a.m. - 5:00 p.m. (EST). E-mail address: docdelivery@haworthpress.com].

http://www.haworthpress.com/web/JHASO
© 2004 by The Haworth Press, Inc. All rights reserved.
Digital Object Identifier: 10.1300/J187v03n01_08

December 27, 2003 and January 17, 2004 I interviewed by telephone 6 colleagues, living in various parts of the U.S. These respondents are all "out" about having HIV, accustomed to advocacy and public speaking, and eager to expand their audience to perhaps give service providers more insight into the needs, experiences, and strengths of older people living with HIV. These participants range in age from 53 to 68, and the time they have been living with HIV is from 10 to 20 years.

These 6 vignettes were developed from notes I took during one-time telephone conversations ranging from 45 to 90 minutes. I told each participant I was interested in their experiences living with HIV; their thoughts and feelings regarding being middle-aged or older; and the intersection of AIDS and aging, as if they were on a panel in front of service providers. I asked them what name to use and what demographic characteristics they wished to share, then invited them to say anything they wished about growing older with HIV. During this project I tried to act as a journalist, doing a verbatim documentation. The interviews were not tape-recorded. I took notes on the computer as they spoke, and direct quotes are from these notes. Sometimes I have grouped related comments together for coherence. Anything in { }'s is a clarification or definition inserted into the participant's account. I sent each individual summary to the relevant person for a check for accuracy and appropriateness. After each account was finalized and with everyone's verbal request and permission, I sent the entire draft article to each interviewee before it was submitted for publication.

The participants differ in aged, gender, ethnicity, region, sexual orientation, history, time of knowing their HIV diagnosis, and method they think they were infected, but it seems that living with HIV over 50 has led to several commonalities in their lives. Everyone brought up the subjects of support, stigma, activism, health maintenance, the difficulty of separating the effects of HIV from the effects of aging, and a renewed gratitude about life and love. I was moved by how forthcoming all of these participants were about their own mortality and about the preciousness of life. They honored me by speaking their truths without flinching. I encourage you to read these accounts carefully and in their entirety, with an open mind and heart. These "panelists" have eloquently articulated their experiences because they wanted to help us to help other HIV-infected older persons.

SUSAN:
"I DON'T KNOW WHAT IT'S LIKE TO GROW OLDER WITHOUT HIV."

Susan identified herself as a 53-year-old straight White woman. She now lives in Aiken, SC, which is where she was raised. She believes that she became infected when she was dating her future husband. She and her husband had not been married long when he became very ill. She learned in September

1987 that she had HIV, 11 days after her husband learned that he had AIDS. He was diagnosed with PCP {pneumosistis carinii pneumonia} and HIV, and his T-cell count was 34. She remembers vividly that he was getting 12 AZT pills a day, and the anemia that resulted required repeated blood transfusions. He lived for two years after his diagnosis. The last six months he was very impaired, and in the last two months he was bedridden with encephalitis. Susan's physical condition was also frail: she qualified for disability and stopped working. For five years after her husband's death, Susan was very active as a volunteer and public speaker in Columbia, the state capital. Then she moved back to her hometown, where she has lived a quieter life for the last 9 years, enjoying the grandson that she almost didn't live to see.

Susan gave this account of her activism soon after our conversation began: "For five years I was on a crusade to educate people. I was bound and determined to keep HIV from happening to other people. I was totally driven by the need to prevent infection. My message was: 'It happened to me and it can happen to you.' Then I stopped public speaking because I felt like I was repeating myself–my story never changed, of course–and even though I was reaching some people, I felt like it wasn't doing that much good. Plus, when I moved back to Aiken in 1996, I was on the verge of getting sick and I started taking P.I.'s {protease inhibitors} and didn't know what effect they would have on me. I felt like I was coming home to be near my family and to die. My energy level was bad, my t-4 count was low, and my viral load was high, and I just pulled in. I thought that was where my journey was taking me, that I wouldn't live but a couple more years. So I stopped being public and got more private."

She attributes her survival to the new medication options: "I probably wouldn't have lived this long if it weren't for the P.I.'s I started taking around 1996. Suddenly my viral load went to undetectable and I had more energy. The P.I.'s are the reason I'm here now. That's why I'm still alive, and still healthy. The last 7 years were a gift. I'm just thrilled. Things couldn't be better. I'm capable of living a normal life now; I work full-time. I'm at a very good place in my life. I'm so lucky; my needs are so few right now."

Susan brought up the devastation of HIV discrimination: "The stigma is a big deal. That's what makes this disease so hard, in addition to the physical struggles. When I tested positive, there was such a stigma about HIV that it didn't matter how you got it–you still had shame and guilt. In general, people are nice to my face, but you never know what they say when you're not there. I've only been blackballed once, and that was in 1992 from extended family members who didn't want me on vacation with them because I had HIV, and they let me know that. I went anyway! That's the only time it ever hit me head on. I was lucky because I'm White, attractive, educated, straight, married, and middle-class. I've faced no stigma except for HIV. I think I got special treatment for my being in a position of privilege in society. People would see me as an 'innocent victim' and that would really tick me off; fighting that idea was part of my crusade. I didn't see myself as a victim at all and I never blamed my husband; he never sought this disease and he didn't mean to give it to me. I kept telling people that it doesn't matter how anyone gets it. I didn't want to play into the prejudice toward Gay men and drug users. I know that was part of what made my talks effective; people had stereotypes about who got this illness, and I blew their stereotypes to bits."

Susan commented on the importance of stable social support: "I've been very lucky; my close friends are still my close friends. Everyone on my job knows, and my family members know." She didn't always have the support she wanted from family, however. When she tested positive, a sister begged her not to tell their mother. "I would have loved to have support from my mom, but she died without knowing that I had HIV. She thought my husband died of leukemia. My sister didn't want my mom to know, and I honored her wishes."

Susan spoke of several ways in which having HIV changed her life: "HIV made my world smaller, but that was on purpose, because my priorities changed. I have no patience for being around people who aren't important to me or who don't share my values. I don't know if this is because of HIV, or being older, or both. The biggest loss from having HIV has been that I haven't had a partner, and that wasn't on purpose. I miss having companionship; I miss having a grandpa for my grandson. I know there are people with HIV who find partners after they test positive, but that hasn't happened for me. That has caused some pain for me in the past. Now my work and family and home take all of my attention and energy, and that loss is less significant."

When asked about growing older as a HIV-positive woman, Susan immediately commented on how fortunate she feels: "I sure am older than I expected to get. There are rarely bad days for me emotionally, because every day is a blessing. I'm so grateful not only to just *be here*, but to have my children and grandchild."Age has even brought advantages: "I don't know what it would be to be my age and just find out I had HIV. But having lived with it for over 16 years, I'm doing OK. HIV is easier for me in every way than when I was young. I'm more content with myself and my life. I've always tried to make the best of whatever, but with age has come more wisdom and contentment."

As she reflected on the intersection of HIV with aging, she said: "I don't know what it's like to grow older without HIV. I don't have a comparison. I don't have a 'me' that matured without having HIV. It's been a part of my life for almost half of my adult life. I was diagnosed at 36. Now I'm 53. HIV has been there for so long. I do sometimes wonder–if I woke up tomorrow and there was a cure, would it really make a difference in my life? HIV is so much a part of my life now." Then she laughed and added, "Of course, it's easy to have this positive attitude when you're well; I don't know how I would be talking if I were really sick. Whenever I feel bad, I always wonder 'is this the one I won't recuperate from?' It's always such a relief to get back to 'normal' again–that is, what's normal for my body."

She talked about her financial situation: "My biggest thought about surviving this long is that I have the same worries every other single woman my age does when they aren't financially secure–practical worries that I didn't think I would have. I used to spend money like crazy and go on trips back when I didn't think I was going to live. Now I'm living–which is wonderful-but I need to be careful and plan for life rather than death. I have a little nest egg, but not enough to retire."

She has learned over the years to attend to her health, but cannot separate the effects of HIV from the effects of aging: "I really take good care of myself. I listen to my body. If it gets tired, I stop. I get lots of sleep, I exercise, and I don't drink or smoke. But who knows? I may have taken good care of myself because I'm growing older. Are these changes in my behavior due to HIV or due to age?"

She reflected on what meant the most to her in the early years when she first knew she was infected: "The women's support group I was in was the best thing that ever happened to me. We all got HIV in different ways, but we all felt the same way. That really increased my ability to cope with it. The support group made me more aware that all the shame and stigma I felt was not unusual. That made a lot of difference in my life."

Susan is not connected to an AIDS Service Organization or support group: "I haven't searched for a support group or ASO here {in Aiken}, but I have recently begun to realize that I'm feeling a little isolated. Sometimes I long to find someone who understands people with HIV. I probably need a professional individual who has empathy, background, and knowledge. I guess I need that more than I admit to myself. I am thinking about volunteering again, to help others with HIV. That's a form of therapy for me. I've been through all the ups and downs and ins and outs; I've lived with this for over 16 years and I know what's what. I don't need support for myself as much as I need to help others."

I asked what she would say to social workers and other service providers; she replied: "I would tell social workers that their work is invaluable. When I think of my journey of the last 16 or 17 years, the social workers stand out in my mind as being the most helpful. It's so important to have someone you can count on–someone genuine and helpful, someone who knows about the disease and understands how to get you what you need."

Throughout the interview Susan insisted that she was doing OK. I leave you with these words: "HIV has turned my life around in some ways, in good ways. Life is good, that's all I can say. I have such peace and serenity. I'm just glad to be here."

SHIRLEY:
"LIFE COULD HAVE PUT YOU
ON THIS SIDE OF THE DESK."

Shirley identified as a 55-year-old African-American Lesbian. She lives in Dorchester, MA. A former intravenous drug user, she is not sure whether she was infected through sharing syringes or through unprotected sex. In the early 1980's, there was little information about how HIV was transmitted, and the word wasn't getting out to drug users or women. She had been in recovery from drug use for 7 years before the HIV test became available in 1985. She took the test right away and learned she was infected. She has known of her HIV status for almost 19 years, and may have been infected for 26 years. She considers herself a long term survivor.

Shirley counts herself lucky that she recovered from her drug use, which she thinks could have killed her long ago: "When my mother died when I was 14, my whole life changed. I was angry at her, because she left me with two brothers to raise, and deal with my father, who expected me to run the house. Recovery was the best thing that ever happened to me. I stopped medicating that pain and anger. If I hadn't come in from the street, I would have died. I was real clear that I wasn't going to use drugs again. I never relapsed, even through all this stress of testing HIV-positive and thinking I was going to die. Now I'm that same 14-year-old frightened girl who has become a 55-year-old women who has support. Pieces were missing in the building blocks of my life, and I had to go back and put it back together myself."

She described the early days of the epidemic, when it was difficult to get accurate and timely information: "As a Black Lesbian, I wasn't getting *any* information. During that time, there was little information about it, and there were no support systems, no educational opportunities. They were still trying to figure out what caused this disease. People who were dying were saying it was 'bad blood.' We didn't even realize in the beginning it came from sharing needles. We were told it affected only Gay White men."

She recounts the turmoil and hopelessness of testing positive: "The reason I got tested was I was getting into a relationship with someone I cared a great deal about and my life had changed for the better. It was a shock to test positive, but it was not unexpected, because I had not protected myself in any way. When I tested positive my doctor of 6 years told me that she didn't have any experience with this, didn't want to deal with it, couldn't give me any information, and couldn't refer me anywhere. She said that there was nothing that could be done, and that I should go home and get my affairs in order. I knew people who were dying fast of this disease; I really expected to pass away. During that early time, every little cough, every sore, every little fever, I just expected that that would be the end, the downward spiral, because we didn't know. It was a horrible time. And I didn't know what would happen to my kids; I had no extended family."

She is very enthusiastic about doing public speaking: "I speak at forums, schools, and transitional living programs, and I tell people about my early years and the consequences of not having support. I tell everyone that whatever decisions you make today will come back on you tomorrow, so get support for your decision making today. Community support is the only way that people can learn, grow, and change. My positive attitude came from trial and error, the school of hard knocks, I didn't just wake up one morning with this view. That's why I try to use my experience to help others. Not to browbeat them, but to say what my life was like. People don't come with instructions; you have to figure out how to get what you need in order to function."

Shirley is a firm believer in asking for help: "I had a lot of support for the first two years, and I was able to get through it only because of that. Right after I tested positive I found a support group for women who were terminally ill, and I got a great deal of support from them. I was the only woman of color, and the only poor woman, and the only woman with HIV, but still I was able to use it to my benefit. And I told my Lesbian support group about having HIV, because my recovery was all about getting support from people."

It was initially hard for her to get support, but then the situation improved: "Since the recovery community didn't know it was passed through needles, they weren't supporting people with HIV. But after two years I began to find people with HIV in the recovery community. In the third year I found a recovery group for people with HIV. This was a mixed group–men, women, Gays, straights–it came out of a common need. The fourth year, I found a health center that had a women of color with HIV support group. That was a gift from heaven. Close, connective, lifelong friendships were formed there. There were women in different stages of dying, and women in different stages of living. There were different strengths you could learn from. There were positives and negatives that you could use to learn from."

She also experienced a down side to having a strong personal support network: "Even though I got support from people, they also caused me stress, because I had to take care of them as well. They were stressed because they cared about me. I felt like I had to make sure that they were OK. I got closer than I was before with my friends, but I got to the point where I had to push them away. There was nothing to support them either. The families and lovers didn't get support at that time."

I asked her how things changed over time as she lived with HIV. She said, "The first two years was a process of seeking help, and when I realized that there was nothing else I could do, I let go of the worry. The second year, I realized that I wasn't just going to drop dead–there was new information that people were living longer. And I had to remember that my kids were my responsibility and I had to do the best for them." She still wants to take good care of her family: "I use my support groups to make sure that I don't put stress on my family. I want their lives to be as normal as I can make it. I want to take care of them. And when I can't do it, I feel like I'm letting people down. But I try to be real with people, to let them know what I can and cannot do. There's no pretense here–I can do what I can do, and I am who I am."

She had a hard time with the idea that she might leave her kids without a mother: "When I learned I was HIV-infected, my daughter was around 14, and I felt like I was doing to her what my mother had done to me. I put a lot of stress on her; I didn't tell my children I had HIV because I didn't want them to worry.

I told my daughter when she was 18 and in the Coast Guard. She told me she already knew! She had overheard me on the telephone several years ago and was waiting for me to tell her. Now the kids are ages 33 and 25. I thought I would be leaving them, but I lived to see them grown. They are wonderful, caring people. They are great, and I'm so lucky."

Shirley spontaneously spoke of living with stigma: "I was ashamed of being uneducated, of being promiscuous, of using drugs. Then HIV on top of all that. I felt ashamed, and I wondered why God would do this to me. Now, usually I am completely out about who I am, including my HIV. But I'm not *always* out about HIV because I don't always feel safe. I still fear the judgements that people still put on you, that you got the virus because you did something wrong, and on top of that you're old. The stigma is elevated when you're over 50, because people don't think of you as being sexual. 'Oh, this old lady got AIDS?' There's a stigma about age, and judgements about age. All the uncertainties of fearing that people will reject you."

I asked what was different about being middle-aged: "Living with the virus as you get older makes you take better care of yourself, you take stock of yourself and clarify what's important. I still go to support groups. I have friends and comrades that I talk to about the virus. And I take care of myself with massages and acupuncture. Today the skills I learned in the early years help me get through. Some days I don't think about it. But some days I stay in bed all day with body pain and mental pain. But I've learned to let someone know when I'm having a bad day. I call friends and talk about life, about living, about the recipe for living. It brings me back to reality."

She sees having HIV as a mixed bag: "I'm lucky because I've lived a long time with this virus. I haven't been in the hospital or had any opportunistic infections; my t-cells are good and my viral load is undetectable. But it's still stressful to have this illness. Sometimes I grieve for myself, I feel sorry for myself, I feel such a sense of loss, having this virus. But then I realize the good parts: meeting wonderful people, going to the schools talking to kids, being self-motivated. I wouldn't have those things if it weren't for HIV."

Shirley rejoices at growing older: "I didn't expect to get this old. When I turned 50, it was quite a blessing. Turning 50 was wonderful, because it was quite an achievement. I took a look at my life and said, 'this is not so bad. I don't have to lie to people, I don't put on airs, I feel good most days, I have a loving relationship.' About being 55–I'm loving it. Every day is a blessing. I've lived with this virus for a long time. I didn't just get it. I'm older, I can decide what I want, what I don't want."

However, she also notices a fading of physical stamina with age: "The downside of growing older is you don't have the energy and strength you had when you were younger, so normal aches and pains are exacerbated. Issues as we age are more critical. Regular illnesses are more elevated in their effects, not only because I'm getting older, but also because of the virus. Sometimes I don't know whether it's HIV or aging."

She still struggles at times financially, but she feels very fortunate: "I'm very lucky–I have a car, I have a home. I'm on disability, but I'm not desperate. I'm very careful about spending money."

Shirley commented on the ongoing struggle with being on antiretrovirals: "Every day when I get up to take my pills, I'm still dealing with this issue. I hate taking the pills, but that's part of the day, like taking a shower. The pills are always a reminder. When you deal with something so long, it's a reminder that this virus is never going to go away. There are things I would like to do that I'll never be able to do because of the side effects, like short term memory loss, low grade fevers, and diarrhea, so I can't go back to school like I want to. But I've learned not to spend time worrying about when I'm going to die. I'm going to live as long as I can live. That's the positive that I put on myself. And that's what I tell other people."

She feels HIV as a sword hanging over her head: "There are still uncertain times, wondering when and how I'm going to get ill. Every time I have a severe cold, I think 'is this the pneumonia that will take me away?' When I have a pain in my side, I think 'is this liver failure?' Being over 50 and knowing that I won't bounce back like I used to–that's a worry."

She had this message for social workers: "I have experienced judgement from professionals. What I want social workers to know is we're people like you. Because you're sitting behind that desk, it doesn't make you any better than me. Don't put a judgement on me just because I'm asking for help. Life could have put you on this side of the desk." She also recommended that we work in true partnership: "When I got the virus, there was nobody to help me. Now there are services, but I am still fighting through attitudes and red tape. I have a right to make my own decisions, but service providers sometimes think they have the right to make decisions for you; they dis-empower you. I think that people think that when you get HIV, you get stupid! They want to decide what you should do and how. But they're not living with this virus, every day, every day."

Shirley ended by acknowledging that there were many helpers who were genuinely interested and effective: "I think that there are a lot of nice people out there, looking for information on how to really help people. I'm really glad to be able to share my experiences with them, because I know their hearts are in the right place."

TOM:
"IT'S LIKE AN EARTHQUAKE. HOW CAN YOU BLAME YOURSELF FOR A BOULDER FALLING ON YOU?"

Tom identified himself as a 68-year-old White Gay man. He lives in Brooklyn, NY. He believes he contracted HIV through sex with men. He had always felt that he didn't need to know his HIV status because he wasn't convinced there were any treatments that would help. Then in 1995 he landed in the hospital with PCP, and was diagnosed with AIDS. He thinks he may have been infected for about 10 years.

He told the story of his diagnosis in this way: "I was in the hospital with PCP when I was 60, and that's how I was diagnosed with AIDS. The diagnosis was no great surprise. I knew I was in a risk category, but I didn't take the test because there was not much hope for treatment. At the time, I didn't even want to know. GMHC {Gay Men's Health Crisis} had said that if you don't know how you're going to react, don't get a test. I heard and believed that. Knowing your status didn't do you any good. I didn't want AZT, so I didn't get tested. I may have been infected for 10 years. I'm not curious about it; the length of time is not relevant. I care about how much longer I have to live, not the past."

Tom finds much meaning in telling his story to others: "I've done a lot of public speaking. For 8 years, ever since I found out. It gives me purpose, it gets me out, it gives me something to do. And in telling others, you have to figure out what your core is, what you really believe. You have to focus. So in that respect it's good for me too. It's healthy for me to go out and talk about this. I get to address the big questions; I can't escape them; I have to be truthful about it. I don't want to be locked up in the prison of stigma and secrecy. Doing things is better than sitting there and thinking 'woe is me.'"

He said another reason he is open about HIV is that he doesn't want to contribute to stigma: "The more people who are open, the less stigma comes to others. It's healthier that way. If we hide, it allows stigma to perpetuate. Not everyone likes that, but I've decided to go that way. It's still so secretive. I had a friend who died two months ago, but he never said he had AIDS, although I think it was." When he first knew he was infected he felt the stigma as well: "I felt I needed to put a skull and crossbones on me because I was now poison." He now feels strongly that internalized stigma is debilitating: "I find that people with HIV often blame themselves, and I have a hard time listening to other's guilt. I once had internalized stigma, and I rejected it in myself. I also reject stigma in other people; it's another type of contamination. I stopped going to one support group because of that. I would rather walk away from that. I grew up in Tennessee, and I can no longer tolerate Bible-belt type judgement. HIV is a virus; it's like an earthquake. How can you blame yourself for a boulder falling on you? I'm very concerned about internalized stigma. We need to get past it. It's the biggest danger we have. We need to feel good about ourselves; it will help us live longer and better."

He said that when he learned he has HIV, he viewed life in a completely different way: "I just knew I had to change my life. I buried the person I was before, and became another. It was a conscious act. I thought 'I can no longer live I way I was, that person is dead.' My identity changed. I became more aware of the worthiness of existence, of living a fruitful and productive life. I had to do things differently, with purpose. I could no longer just walk through a field of clover. I was careful and conscious about my life." He copes through having a varied identity and activities: "I'm part of the larger world, not just the HIV world. That's very important to me. I'm in a group of older people as well. What I do has to do with *life*."

Reflecting on the intersection of HIV and aging, Tom said: "I don't know what the terrain would have been if I had been younger when I got it; I may have died. I have more coping skills than I had before; that's an advantage of being older. They say older people are wiser; I don't know if that's true. But I do know that my adherence to medication is so much better at my age than when I would have been when I was younger. I never miss a pill. Older people don't have the luxury of making mistakes any more; our mistakes are more costly. Young people think they're immortal, but I know I'm not."

Tom reports both benefits and drawbacks to the anti-HIV medications: "I feel lucky. I'm glad to be alive; I could have died and I didn't. When I came out of the hospital, within 3 months, HAART {highly active antiretroviral therapy} appeared. If I had gotten sick a year earlier, I wouldn't have had the same chances. I know the medicine has kept me alive. It's part luck, and it's part science. I know that therapies are getting better, and I could continue to live a long time. My viral load is undetectable, and has been for a while. But the protocols are like navigating through a mine field. I have serious neuropathy and diabetes, both brought on by antiretrovirals. I'm on insulin twice a day."

He remarked on the importance of social services: "In the hospital they gave me a referral to a group for persons over 50 with HIV. I also saw a social worker there. She and the group got me through the danger–the physical and psychological danger." Tom wants social workers to know this: "All people with HIV need some emotional help, although they may not ask for it. It's a mental stress. The most difficult part for social workers is knowing that someone has the virus; most people don't want to disclose that they are infected. You must get to know them and engage them and make it safe for them to tell you. I think social workers are the most adept at this. The person has to trust the social worker; you have to have a place and person where you will be responded to in a caring manner. Some places react negatively to the virus; people with HIV have a sixth sense–we can detect the animosity or hostility, and we avoid it. I don't go where I don't feel safe. Most people will do the same. I think that depression and loneliness is the biggest threat to our mental health, as we isolate ourselves more and more. Our friends are dying from HIV, cancer, and age. Our social network is diminishing. The biggest challenge is not being alienated. We need to keep the will to live. My message is: nurture the will to live. It's so easy to give up, and to toss yourself figuratively out the window. Social workers should let people with HIV use the strength already within them."

MARY: "I NEVER EXPECTED TO GET TO THIS AGE."

Mary defines herself as a 66-year-old Latina mother, grandmother, and great grandmother. Mary's grandparents were from Mexico and her parents were both born in Texas. Mary was born and raised in Austin, where she still lives. From birth to age six, she lived in a Catholic orphanage and then went to live with her parents. She remains Catholic, and raised her children in that tradition as well. Mary was infected through blood transfusions she received during surgery in 1984. She found out in 1987 that she has HIV when she was contacted by a blood bank that was notifying people who received HIV-infected blood. Then she suddenly understood the weeks of flu-like symptoms she suffered shortly after her surgery three years earlier. She said: "1987 was the year I got my master's degree, the year my mother-in-law died, and the year I learned I had HIV."

Mary gets a lot of meaning from her life as an advocate. She has been completely open about her HIV status since 1992, when she was asked by a union representative to do a cover story in the union magazine to educate the public employees about HIV. She said, "I felt like I was supposed to do this" and did not hesitate. Since that time she has devoted herself to public speaking. She has traveled all over the world, including Japan, to talk about her experience with HIV. She has 12 binder notebooks–titled "my journey with HIV"–filled with her speeches, conferences, and appearances. She said: "Every opportunity I get, I do education, for free. I always incorporate my own diagnosis, so they know they know someone with HIV."

Her most notable activism effort was her 1994 court case against the city of Austin after they pressured her to quit her job with them. "I lost my job in 1992 when I went public about having HIV; my boss and co-workers harassed me so much that my doctor advised me to leave because the stress was making me sick. I didn't want to leave because that was my only source of health insurance. I said 'I have a right to work' but my doctor asked me if my job was worth losing my health. So I decided to quit and sue the city. The lawsuit was very painful to me. People at work, people I'd been friends with for 12 years, testified against me. But it was worth it overall, because I won the first HIV discrimination court case in Austin. Mine was the only HIV discrimination case they didn't settle out of court. I never wanted to settle out of court, even if it was for more money; I wanted my case on the record, for other attorneys to be able to find as a precedent." The jury awarded her money and said that the city had to hire her back; but the city refused. "They delayed their decision for two years; they were waiting for me to die, but I fooled them [laughs]."

Also in 1994 she co-founded with a social worker a women's HIV group because she felt the need to be with other women, but hadn't been able to find a group. These days she's an advisory member. They continue to meet, and periodically sponsor conferences called "HIV university" to learn about treatment updates.

Mary said that she has been quite disturbed by HIV stigma: "It doesn't matter how you got the virus, it matters what you do after you know you have it. When I first tested positive, I could never understand the stories of betrayal that I heard. Parents who threw their children out. Sadly enough, the stigma has not yet gone away. Even though people don't talk about it as much anymore, it's still there." She says that through her public speaking she notices "ignorance about HIV at every educational level and age group. Stigma is still there; it's everywhere." She recounted fighting her local Catholic church over an incident where several persons with HIV were invited to a meeting to talk about helping people with HIV, only to be asked immediately and rudely to leave. In a protest letter to the bishop she said: "We only need three things: love, understanding, and compassion."

She reflected on the effect of age on HIV stigma: "It's especially difficult for older people to come out about being infected. As an older person you're supposed to be the example; you're not supposed to have any faults. And HIV seems like a fault, because people blame you for having it. The first thing that goes through people's mind is that you used drugs or had unprotected sex or were careless."

Mary says she is in relatively good health, although she has had some major struggles. She had a mild stroke 5 years ago, caused by HIV. She had been taking 12 or 13 pills a day, but recently went off all medications because of anemia, diarrhea, and weight loss. She has some neuropathy and arthritis in one hand. She says she's in good shape now "for my age and having HIV." When asked about growing older, she said the only difference she has noticed is not having the energy she used to have.

She asked her doctor recently for a prognosis, because she's had HIV for 20 years and had been reading that she was probably at the upper limit of survival for persons with HIV. Her doctor replied that he considers Mary a long-term survivor, and believes that Mary could live long enough to die of an age-related illness. She is grateful and amazed. She keeps sight of the frailty and uncertainty of life, and strives to make sure that she organizes her legacies for her children. Last year she made photo albums for them all; this year she is putting together a family history so they don't lose her knowledge of their roots.

Mary has felt much support from the younger generations in the family, especially her 5 children. The older grandchildren all know she has HIV; many of them have walked with her on AIDS walks. Her 44-year marriage is possibly her greatest source of sustenance. Recently her husband has developed some health problems of his own: he has diabetes, and had a light stroke. He was disturbed at his illnesses, because he had been seeing himself primarily in the role of Mary's caregiver, not the other way around. Mary told him "how about if we take care of each other?" Of her husband, she said: "Whatever time we have together is a blessing. We enjoy each other, the kids, and life. We feel fortunate that we've gotten this far. We live a full life."

She is very concerned about older persons and prevention: "The older people really need to be educated about HIV and treatment. Older people aren't aware that they should be careful, that they should use condoms. Older people don't realize they are susceptible. Especially Latinas, especially if they're Catholic, don't use condoms. Retired women, especially in congregate settings, don't realize that one man may be dating several women. Seniors are dying to know; who's going to tell us? Not our doctors, not our children. We have to educate each other. To this day, this isn't being addressed adequately. But how do you get older people together when their energy isn't what it once was?" She thinks that HIV education should be done in congregate and residential settings. She suggests that older men and women should be separated for HIV education; they'll be more afraid to talk openly if they're together. She suggested that the HIV session be nested in a series of health workshops–start with conditions like diabetes and heart conditions, and discuss HIV after people are used to each other.

She had this message for service providers: "Social workers need to take the blinders off their eyes and realize that older people do get HIV. They think we don't have sex lives. Please look at us as we really are."

Of her 20 years with HIV she says: "I feel that it's been a spiritual journey. I feel that God has a plan for me; I just don't know what it is." Mary is deeply grateful that she has lived so long with HIV, and rejoices in having lived this long with her family: "This February, I will mark 20 years of having HIV. We're celebrating my survival. I feel so lucky to have my grandchildren. I feel really blessed; there were so many things I didn't know I'd be around for; I never expected to get to this age. I want to enjoy life every day, day by day, every day is an extra gift; I don't want to waste my time in regrets or 'what ifs.'" Her message to everyone is: "Live today as if today's your last day, and you'll enjoy it more, you won't complain as much."

JIM:
"HAVING HIV IS A LONG, SLOW PROCESS. IT'S LONGER THAN PEOPLE'S ATTENTION SPAN."

Jim identified himself as a 58-year-old Gay White man of Irish Catholic descent. He lives in Cambridge, MA, which is where he was raised. He believes he was infected in the 1980s through sex with men. In 1989 his lover, with whom he had a long-term monogamous relationship, died from AIDS. At that time Jim assumed that he too was infected. Because there was no proven treatment, he saw no reason to take the HIV test. However, in 1992 he decided that he wanted to know where he was medically, wanted to know his T-cell count, because he was curious about his prognosis. He explained, "I was running out of money and wanted just to know how much longer I had to live."

He recounted how difficult emotionally it was to receive confirmation of his HIV status: "Even being relatively sure I was positive, it was hard for me to go back to get the results. I put it off a few weeks. I didn't want to hear it. Once I heard it, it took me another few months to figure out what I was going to do about medical care. It took months to adjust, to start to deal with it. It was a time when people were dying in an ugly way–wasting, Kaposi's Sarcoma–and there were times when one thought about suicide as an option. It was bleak."

Jim brought up his concern with the continued stigma around HIV: "I see stigma all the time, in all communities, even the Gay community. There's lots of separatism. The HIV community stays to itself, with their own groups. It's another form of segregation. Stigma is always there, even if it's in the form of self-blame. No matter how you got it, HIV makes you 'less than' because now you need a case manager, you need help. People don't talk about this enough, that we aren't 'less than' just because we have HIV."

Jim decided from the beginning not to hide his diagnosis: "I was always open about having HIV. It's a virus. I'm not ashamed of having it. I would rather not have gotten it, but I never felt like I was second class. But I'm also a White middle class male and was therefore more accepted. And as a Gay male, I was part of a larger group. I wasn't as stigmatized as some, like those of color or poor or on drugs."

Jim explained that being HIV-infected becomes a person's major concern: "HIV is such a huge part of my life, just coping with the disease and doctor's appointments and social security–all the bureaucracy that runs your life. HIV really is the center of my life. Having HIV is a full time job. It zaps you of your energy, your cognitive skills, so you don't feel like communicating or taking care of yourself. "

Jim further described the very difficult struggle with living with HIV in one's body: "I've been living with the knowledge that I have HIV for 15 years. There's always a sense that you're alone, no matter what. You may have a peer group, friends, providers, and a lover, but when you close the door, it's *your* body that's failing you. There's a kind of despair and hypochondria that comes with HIV. Even when you're doing well and your counts are good, you never know when your body is going to fail."

As Jim lived longer with HIV, he noticed a lessening of overt support from HIV-negative members of his network: "When I first told people I was infected, they rallied around me. But when I didn't die, people stopped asking me how I am. It feels like others are denying my being sick. People stop asking about how you're feeling, how the tests were, what's happening. It's a non-conversation with family and friends. People know that I go to the doctors, but they don't ask what happens. I think that's not uncommon. I think other people's family members are like this as well–they don't know how to ask. And people have the kind of attention span where they react to emergencies, and having HIV is a long, slow process. It's longer than people's attention span. When I tell family members about a symptom, they remember that I'm infected and they look sad and worried, and I think, 'Oh. I shouldn't have said that.' I'm guarded about what I say. Only my peers–infected peers–really ask me how I am. It's either/or with family members–you're either very sick, or you're well. But my peers can understand the grey areas. We all live in a grey area of our lives; you don't know what you're going to face."

Jim was honest about the overwhelming concern he has for his own survival: "I have very strong and partnering providers–if I didn't, I would move and find someone who would work with me. But it's still hard. You worry for yourself. I've had a bad few months–with lots of friends dying and sick–and it is reminding me that I'm also going to go. I think about my own death."

However, he is quick to speak of the benefits of living with HIV: "There are also great opportunities to meet remarkable people doing remarkable work. That's very rewarding, to sit at a table with people who are making differences in people's lives in a real way, an honest way. Activism does that for me. My priorities got straightened out, and I now tend to meet people who have the same values and priorities I have, and that's a really nice thing. People really think about what they're doing, they're respectful. That's a wonderful way to be. If it weren't for HIV as a life-altering experience, I wouldn't necessarily have met some of the people I've met and been inspired by. There is a blessing there, somewhere. I'm glad my priorities changed. I'm so glad that I'm now trying to make a difference in people's lives."

In some ways, he sees age as irrelevant to a person with HIV: "I'm not sure there are any differences in having HIV, no matter how old you are. The disease is the common ground." He commented that aging and HIV can both reinforce a realignment of priorities: "As you get older, you get to cut through the bull shit. But HIV also helps you cut through the bullshit." He compared HIV and aging in this way: "HIV is like a preparation for getting older, because your body is falling apart with HIV, and that's similar to aging. You tend to lose your peer group to death, and that's similar to aging. With both HIV and aging, you tend to learn how to make and keep friends." He did notice some changes in his perspective as he has entered middle age: "As I age, I don't get as flustered, I don't worry as much, I've learned to roll with the punches. My perspective on aging has changed; I don't worry about wrinkles. And I really appreciate my friends who are dying, who are grateful and full of joy for our time together."

Fearing that he was sounding too dire, he said, "I don't mean to sound pessimistic; I mean to sound honest. There isn't enough said about what it's like to live with HIV. We've forgotten. Service providers have gotten complacent. People look healthier. We haven't really articulated well what it's like to live with a terminal and chronic condition. We've glamorized HIV a little. When we do public speaking, we don't tend to talk about the day-to-day inconvenience and hassles of living with HIV. Kids do think it can be managed with a pill, and that it's 'only a virus.' But HIV is life-altering, and life-threatening."

He wanted to say this to service providers: "Learn to listen. There's a lot that can be taught to providers by PWA's {persons with AIDS}. Everyone is different. Be respectful of all the challenges in everyone's lives. HIV is sometimes the least of someone's problems, because they're also battered, or homeless, or drug addicted. Just listen, because lots of times people are asking for help, and don't know how or where to get it."

KAREN: "I WENT FROM DYING TO LIVING."

Karen is a 57-year-old White widow who believes that she was infected by her husband. She lives in a small rural town in the Midwest. When she was growing up, her family traveled around the world with her military father. She didn't want to specify her location or use her real name because: "I'm out about having HIV, but I'm not out to everyone." Karen's husband of 12 years became ill in 1994 and subsequently tested positive for HIV; his t-4 count was very low. That prompted her taking a test, and she learned she was infected as well. She remembers well the shock of testing positive: "I couldn't believe it was happening; I was married, working, and raising children. I didn't suspect my husband was having sex on the side. He didn't know he had HIV until he got sick." When she tested she was asymptomatic, but had a very suppressed immune system. She went on AZT at that time, then went on combination therapy–including P.I.s–in 1996. She was her husband's primary caregiver until he died in 1999.

She related that in the beginning of this journey she thought she would not live long: "When I first tested positive, I assumed I would die in a year or two. Then the P.I.'s came on board, and I got better. I went from dying to living."

Karen spoke about the challenges of maintaining secrecy in a non-metropolitan area: "Confidentiality is a bigger concern in small towns. People in rural America aren't going to go to their local hospital or health department for testing and treatment, or even to the drug store for prescriptions. They go as far away as they can. I used to drive 45 minutes to another county to get my medicines; now I get them through the mail. I know HIV-positive people who drive 4 hours just to see doctors who know what they were doing." Karen followed up her confidentiality concerns by talking about stigma: "We need to erase the stigmas around HIV and aging. People are frightened of the stigma. Especially in the straight population, I think, it's not talked about. People are afraid of isolation from the community, being blackballed from activities, having your house burned down, losing friends. It's still risky."

She noticed a marked difference in the way their two families received the news that she and her husband had HIV: "Soon after I was diagnosed, I told my family and friends, and everyone was very supportive. But when my husband told his family, everyone backed away. He didn't get the support that he needed; people he had trusted turned their backs and walked away. My parents, friends, and children are all supportive to this day. When my children were in their 20's, I gave them condoms, and told them 'look at us and remember what can happen.'"

She sought out the support of others with HIV: "We had a large support group in the beginning; now it's a small social gathering that meets occasionally. When people are first diagnosed and sent to us by their doctors, it's great for them to see that we long-term survivors are active and well." I asked her about her use of the phrase "long-term survivor," and she responded that she thinks of herself in that way. She said, "I've been living with HIV for ten years; it's now a part of me. You learn to adapt and survive, if you are going to survive. I'm not happy about having HIV, but I've made the attitude shift. You must realize that you still have a life and you can go on, in spite of everything. I relate it to a person crossing a bridge–some make it over, and some don't. Some go backwards, physically and emotionally, but some go forward. I'm going forward."

Karen is active as a public speaker because she feels strongly about the need for HIV prevention: "I have always done a lot of public speaking to the junior and high schools about safer behavior. Now that I'm over 50, I speak a lot to older people about protecting themselves." Deciding to come out publicly was linked to her own education journey: "When I tested positive, I didn't have a clue about HIV. I used to ask my Gay male friends if they were O.K., but I didn't realize I was a risk. Once I had enough information about HIV, about a year later, I started speaking to groups."

Through her speaking engagements she has realized that it is difficult for older persons to acknowledge the need to be safer: "Older people, especially partnered people, don't believe they are at risk. It's frustrating; people are still not realizing the risk. Many older people are divorced or widowed, and on the dating scene, and don't protect themselves." She feels that getting safer behavior messages to older persons may be a unique challenge: "The older generation never grew up with an openness about sexuality; discussing sex with doctors or even partners is unknown. Sex was private."

Karen commented that young people are also not embracing the message as well as she would like: "Young people are very complacent; they think there are good medications and that they can live with HIV without much problem. They don't know that the meds don't always work. Two decades into it, we're still not getting the message out well enough. In the beginning, the gay community did a lot of good education and advocacy, but we've not done much since then. There's a lot of secrecy and denial."

Karen is worried about our failures with HIV prevention: "It's a battle, and I don't know where we're going with it. Are we starting all over again, with another whole generation who aren't protecting themselves? Are we facing drug resistant viruses being spread widely because we're not doing prevention? We're doing some things right, but we're missing a big portion of our audience."

As she reflected on the experience of having HIV as an older person, she said: "The biggest thing is, there's a social isolation that you don't get when you're diagnosed as a young person. The chat rooms on the internet are mostly full of young people. But for those of us over 50, there aren't that many peers to talk to. And if you're living in rural America, you don't discuss it at all."

When asked what the service and advocacy challenges are regarding older people, she responded: "For people who don't know their HIV status, I think we should encourage everyone to get tested; everyone deserves to know their

HIV status; they owe it to themselves. For people who know they have HIV, the challenge is to help them find a good infectious disease doctor, someone who sees others who are older."

She wishes that medical science had more information about what it's like to have HIV in older adulthood: "We need more people doing the research on this age group; and we need more clinical trials for older people with HIV. We need to know about the interactions between HIV medications and medications taken for other conditions common to old age. The body metabolism is different when you're older. So many older people with HIV are living with dual disabilities; they have more than one chronic condition to manage. How does one med affect the other? Is the kidney failure brought about by HIV meds or by aging or genetic reasons? Is the neuropathy caused by HIV or diabetes, and will it get worse? "

Commenting on service provision, she said, "I'm finding that social workers and case managers really aren't asking the questions they need to ask about risk behaviors. Case managers may see you for a gas voucher, but they don't check out whether you have concerns about HIV. I wish they would all talk about prevention and have condoms available, or ask if you have any questions about sex or drug risk. The case managers haven't been trained enough in behavioral risk assessment, and they're uncomfortable discussing people's private behaviors. Case managers are not even prepared to hear or deal with the answers to those questions. Our consortium just had a training on HIV risk, and some case managers walked out because they were uncomfortable with the words we were using." To service providers, she suggested: "You need to get educated, and find your comfort zone, and be able to talk with anyone–young or old–about risk behaviors. You have to be comfortable, because lives are at stake. You have to put aside your personal feelings and look at the big picture."

Her last words to service providers were: "Talk to us. Get yourself educated. So many case managers are detached. Get involved. If an older woman has HIV, embrace her. Help her, because it's hard."

Resource Information:
HIV Over Fifty

Nathan L. Linsk, PhD
and the National Association on HIV Over Fifty

TASK FORCES

National

The National Association on HIV Over Fifty (NAHOF) provides advocacy, education, communication, and support for HIV positive older adults, their families and those who provide care or conduct research on their behalf. NAHOF maintains a newletter and a website, which include an updated version of this resource list, current information, and a bibliography. NAHOF coordinates a network of regional and local groups and a semi-annual meeting provides a national forum on this issue. Contact: Jim Campbell, National Association of HIV Over Fifty, 23 Miner Street, Boston, MA 02115, 617/262-5657, email: nahof@HIVover fifty.org, website: WWW.HIVOVERFIFTY. ORG

Regional and Local

AIDS and Aging Task Force, New Jersey. Contact Daphne Joslin, Department of Community Health, William Patterson College, 300 Pompton Road, Wayne, NJ, 07470, 973-720-2604.

Nathan L. Linsk, PhD, is Professor, Jane Addams College of Social Work, University of Illinois at Chicago.

[Haworth co-indexing entry note]: "Resource Information: HIV Over Fifty." Linsk, Nathan L. Co-published simultaneously in *Journal of HIV/AIDS & Social Services* (The Haworth Press) Vol. 3, No. 1, 2004, pp. 119-122; and: *Midlife and Older Adults and HIV: Implications for Social Service Research, Practice, and Policy* (ed: Cynthia Cannon Poindexter, and Sharon M. Keigher) The Haworth Press, Inc., 2004, pp. 119-122. Single or multiple copies of this article are available for a fee from The Haworth Document Delivery Service [1-800-HAWORTH, 9:00 a.m. - 5:00 p.m. (EST). E-mail address: docdelivery@haworthpress.com].

http://www.haworthpress.com/web/JHASO
Digital Object Identifier: 10.1300/J187v03n01_09

AIDS and Aging Task Force, Miami. Addresses concerns about HIV over 50 in Dade and Monroe Counties. A Senior Action in a Gay Environment chapter has been established as well. Contact Vincent Delgado, 305-576-6611.

Boston Association on HIV Over Fifty. Provides educational programs at conferences and at senior centers, housing developments, extended care facilities of all types and general health agencies. The Association has developed a curriculum to be utilized in the training of HIV/AIDS counselor and other health care professionals. Contact: 617-262-5657.

Chicago Forum on HIV and Aging. Monthly meetings for networking and resource sharing among service providers and those living with HIV. Contact Bill Rydwells, 773-283-0101.

Long Island Association on HIV Over Fifty. Involved in developing symposia and seminars. Contact Terri Banks, imany828@aol.com. Phone 631-225-5500

Los Angeles HIV Over Fifty Group. Weekly meetings at Being Alive, West Hollywood. Contact Keven Kierth, 310-289-2551, ext 16.

New York Association on HIV Over Fifty, Hunter College, New York City. Contact: Kathy Nokes, PhD, Hunter-Bellevue School of Nursing, 425 E. 25th St., NY, NY 10010, 212-481-7594, Kathynokes@aol.com

Northern California Association on HIV Over Fifty. Contact Monica Dea, mdea@psg.ucsf.edu or Paul Quinn, kboyz@mindspring.com, 415-241-9966, 415-597-9308.

SERVICE PROGRAMS

AIDS Case Management, Solano County Health and Social Services Department; Contact: Sue Gusz, 355 Tuolumne St., MS 20-210, Vallejo, CA 94590; Telephone: 707-784-8259.

Area Agency on Aging, Phoenix. Provides AIDS Case mangement under Ryan White CARE for all HIV programs including people over age 50. Contact Debbie Eliot, 1366 East Thomas Rd, #108, Phoenix, AZ 85014; 602-264-2255; FAX: 602-230-9132.

Senior Action in a Gay Environment, New York City. Programs have been funded by Ryan White CARE for case management of HIV+ seniors, and a specialized mental health service. SAGE runs a weekly support group for HIV+ persons over 50. Contact Senior Action in a Gay Environment, 1 Little West 12th Street, 2nd Fl., NY, NY 10011 (212-741-2247).

Senior HIV Intervention Project. This is a two County Senior HIV Intervention Program in Broward and Palm Beach County. This program of education, peer training support groups, referrals, and a resource library has been established to address the needs of older people regarding HIV in one of the nation's most affected areas. Contact: Lisa Agate, Broward County Health Dept, 780 SW 24th Street, Ft. Lauderdale, FL 33315-2613, 954-467-4779.

SUPPORT GROUPS

Elder Family Services, Brooklyn, NY. See above.
The Jeffrey Goodman Special Care Clinic, The Center-L.A. Gay and Lesbian Community Services Center, Los Angeles. Contact: Joni Lavick, M.A., M.F.C.C., Clinical Coordinator, Social Services, The Jeffrey Goodman Special Care Clinic, 1625 N. Schrader Blvd, Los Angeles, CA 90028-9998, 323-993-7500.
Mt. Sinai Hospital Jack Martin Center. A group was established in June of 1993 for HIV+ persons over 50. Contact: Mary Ann Malone, C.S.W., 212-241-0719, Mt. Sinai Medical Center, One Gustave Levy Place, Box 1, New York, NY 10029-6574.

EDUCATIONAL PROGRAMS

Note: Many of the service programs listed above also provide education.

HealthCare Education Associates. HealthCare Education Associates has developed a curriculum, *HIV: What Persons Over 50 Need to Know*, which is used by peer groups in "study circles," and has recently begun development of a curriculum for physicians and other health providers. Contact: Rita Strombeck, Ph. D., HealthCare Education Associates, 1729 East Palm Canyon, Suite A, Palm Springs, CA 92264. Telephone/FAX: 760-323-1784.

VIDEOS

HIV and Older Adults: Age Is No Barrier. Contact NY State AIDS Institute.
HIV/AIDS: It Can Happen to Me. Contact AARP, telephone 202-434-6466.
Older Americans & HIV/AIDS.15-minute instructional video. Contact National Minority AIDS Council http://www.nmac.org/video
The Forgotten Ten Percent. Contact: Rita Strombeck, Ph. D., HealthCare Education Associates, 1729 East Palm Canyon, Suite A, Palm Springs, CA 92264, telephone/FAX: 760-323-1784.
Seniors at Risk: Sex, Drugs and HIV. (28 minutes). Contact telephone 313-567-2251, www.urbansolutions.org

HIV/AIDS and Older Americans. Informational videotape, 7.34 minutes in length, produced as a collaborative project of the Office of AIDS Research, the National Institutes of Health, and the National Minority AIDS Council and designed to be viewed in facilitated group settings. Available free from the National Minority AIDS Council at http://www.nmac.org/video

The Mature Are Not Immune. Videotape produced by Bronx AIDS Services, Inc. Available through Bronx AIDS Services, Inc., 540 East Fordham Road, Bronx, NY 10458, 718-295-5605.

Index

123

For Product Safety Concerns and Information please contact our EU
representative GPSR@taylorandfrancis.com Taylor & Francis Verlag GmbH,
Kaufingerstraße 24, 80331 München, Germany

Batch number: 08164875

Printed by Printforce, the Netherlands